MENTAL DERANGEMENTS IN INDIA

MENTAL DERANGEMENTS IN INDIA

THEIR SYMPTOMS AND TREATMENT

A. W. OVERBECK-WRIGHT

GYAN

Published by

Gyan Publishing House
5, Ansari Road
Daryaganj, New Delhi-110002
Phone: 011-47034999, 9811692060
E-mail: books@gyanbooks.com

Distribution Network
gyanbooks.com
India, USA, Canada, UK, Australia, France

ISBN: 978-81-212-8470-7 (PB)
First Published, 1912

2nd Impression 2023

Printed at: Gyan Press, Delhi.

MENTAL DERANGEMENTS IN INDIA
Author: A. W. OVERBECK-WRIGHT

MENTAL DERANGEMENTS IN INDIA

THEIR SYMPTOMS AND TREATMENT

BEING A HANDBOOK TO

THE THEORY AND PRACTICE OF MENTAL DISEASE IN INDIA TOGETHER WITH NOTES DEALING WITH THE LEGAL ASPECT OF INSANITY AND THE VARIOUS QUESTIONS LIKELY TO ARISE CONCERNING IT

BY

A. W. OVERBECK-WRIGHT

M.B., CH.B., MED. PSYCH. CERT., D.P.H

CAPTAIN, INDIAN MEDICAL SERVICE

CALCUTTA AND SIMLA: THACKER, SPINK & CO

1912

PREFACE.

My object in plunging thus into literature is to give the medical practitioner in India a book which may aid him in his dealings with insanity, give him information as to the various legal proceedings in connection with it, and bring to his notice the latest discoveries as to its causes, for we are now at the commencement of a new era in this respect and every year seems likely to bring forward greater hopes of successfully treating this scourge of humanity in its various forms.

My work makes no pretence of being anything but a compilation, for, though I gained the Medico-Psychological Certificate in 1900 and have worked continuously at this subject ever since, my knowledge is largely gained from books and, except for nearly a year as specialist to the Military Department of the Government of India and the same time as Superintendent of the Agra Asylum, I can only claim about 2 years' practical knowledge gained from time to time in clinical study under my old friend and teacher Dr. Reid of Aberdeen Asylum.

The books consulted mainly in this work are Bruce's "Clinical Psychiatry," and those by Clouston, Bevan Lewis, Maurice Craig, Cræpelin, Berkley, Savage, Mercier and Major Ewens of the Lahore Asylum, and to these authors I would refer any desirous of fuller or more detailed information than is possible in a book of the type I have attempted.

A. W. OVERBECK-WRIGHT.

CONTENTS.

PART I.

CHAPTER I.

MEDICO-LEGAL.

		Page.
I.	ASYLUM OR HOME TREATMENT	2
	Admission into Asylum	3-6, 7
	Detention under observation	6
	Detention pending removal to an asylum ..	7
	Discharge of patients	8-10
	Escape and recapture	10
	Illegal Detention	10
	Certification of patients	8, 11-14
	Transfer of Lunatics to England	14-16
II.	MANAGEMENT OF PROPERTY	16
III.	CRIMINAL RESPONSIBILITY	19
	Criminal Lunatics	22
	Feigned Insanity	23
IV.	TESTAMENTARY CAPACITY	25
V.	CONFIDENTIAL FAMILY ADVICE	27

CHAPTER II.

CAUSATION OF INSANITY.

I.	IDEAS COMMONLY HELD BY THE LAITY AND MANY MEMBERS OF THE MEDICAL PROFESSION ..	29
	The toxic theory of insanity	29
	Macpherson's classification of toxæmias ..	30
	Effects of unstable mental heredity	32
	Manifestation of unstable heredity	32

		Page.
	Child marriages	33
	Effects of consanguineous marriages and the greater stress of modern life	33
	Effects of low vitality	34
II.	EXCITING CAUSES OF INSANITY	34
	Non-toxic	36
	Toxic	37

CHAPTER III.

CLASSIFICATION OF INSANITY.

I.	INSANITIES OF NON-TOXIC ORIGIN	39
II.	INSANITIES OF TOXIC ORIGIN.	
	A. Metabolic Toxæmias	40
	B. Bacterial Toxæmias	41
	C. Alcoholic and Drug Toxæmias	43
III.	NERVOUS DISEASES FREQUENTLY COMPLICATED BY MENTAL DISEASES	44
IV.	STATES OF MENTAL ENFEEBLEMENT	44

CHAPTER IV.

DERANGEMENTS OF MENTALISATION.

Elevation and excitement	45
Mental confusion	45
Hallucinations	46
Illusions	48
Delusions	48
Stupor	49
Mental Enfeeblement	50
Self-control	50
Impulsiveness	51
Attention	51
Sexual Desire	52
Æsthetic and religious instincts	52
Volition	52
Memory	53

	Page.
Speech	53
Incoherence	54
Disturbances of the emotions	54
Jealousy	55
Sleep	56

CHAPTER V.

Physical Derangements.

Alimentary System	60
Hæmopoietic System	61
Circulatory System	64
Respiratory System	64
Integument	65
Urinary System	66
Reproductive System	67
Vasomotor and Nutritional Disturbances	68
Derangements of Nervous System	69
State of pupils	70
State of reflexes	71
Paresis	71
Attention	72

CHAPTER VI.

General Pathology.

I. General remarks on recent research ..	74
Gross lesions and their import	75
Changes in the cranial bones	75
Lesions of the Dura Mater	75
Lesions of the Pia Mater	76
Gross lesions of the brain substance	77
Degeneration of nerve cells	79
Degeneration of nerve fibres	81
Lesions of the neuroglia	82
Lesions of cerebral arteries and veins	82

Page.

II. CLINICAL PATHOLOGY 82
Temperature 83
Bacteria of mouth and stomach 84
Coagulation of blood 84
Hæmolysis 84
Leucocytosis 85
Leucocytosis in Metabolic Toxæmias 86
Leucocytosis in Bacterial Toxæmias 87
Leucocytosis in G. P. I. 90
Leucocytosis in alcoholic and drug toxæmias .. 91
Leucocytosis in Idiots and Imbeciles 91
Common features of all bacterial toxæmias .. 91
Agglutinines 92

CHAPTER VII.

CLINICAL EXAMINATION OF PATIENTS. 93-96

CHAPTER VIII.

BRIEF DISCUSSION OF THE MAIN DIFFERENCES BETWEEN EUROPEAN AND INDIAN PSYCHOSES.

The Influence of a Tropical climate upon Neurotic Individuals 97
Psychoses peculiar to India 98
Differences of incidence and manifestations of Psychoses common to both the East and the West 101

PART II.

CHAPTER IX.

NEURASTHENIC AND HYSTERICAL CONDITIONS.

I. NEURASTHENIA 104
Definition 104
Ætiology 104
Symptomatology 105
Neuromuscular asthenia 105

		Page.
	Insomnia	106
	Mental depression	107
	Headache	108
	Pains in the back	109
	Cardiac disturbances	109
	Digestive troubles	110
	Mental Symptoms	112
	Motor-mental agitation	113
	Neurasthenic anxiety and compulsory Ideas	114
	Diagnosis	115
	Treatment	116
	Hygienic	116
	Dietetic	117
	Moral	118
	Therapeutic	119
	Hydrotherapy	120
	Drugs	120
	Prognosis	121
II.	NEURASTHENIC PSYCHOSES	121
III.	HYSTERICAL PSYCHOSES	122
	Diagnosis from Neurasthenia	122
	Ætiology	123
	Deviations from normal mentalisation proper to hysteria	124
	Interparoxysmal period	124
	Postparoxysmal Psychoses	125
	Suicidal attempts in hysteria	126
	Treatment	126

CHAPTER X.

INSANITIES OF NON-TOXIC ORIGIN.

I.	EXHAUSTION INSANITIES	127
	Ætiology	127
	Symptoms :—Prodromal	127
	Physical	127
	Mental	129

		Page.
	Treatment	130
	Prognosis	131
	Diagnosis	131
II.	INSANITY RESULTING FROM GROSS BRAIN LESIONS	131
III.	TRAUMATIC INSANITY	133
	Ætiology	133
	Physical Symptoms	134
	Mental Symptoms	135
	Diagnosis	136
	Prognosis	136
	Treatment	137
IV.	INSANITY RESULTING FROM BRAIN ANÆMIA ..	138
	Ætiology	138
	Symptoms :—	
	Physical	138
	Mental	139
V.	INSANITY RESULTING FROM DEPRIVATION OF THE SPECIAL SENSES	139
	Treatment	140
	Prognosis	141

CHAPTER XI.

INSANITIES OF TOXIC ORIGIN.

GROUP I.

	INSANITIES DUE TO METABOLIC TOXÆMIAS ..	142
I.	ACUTE MELANCHOLIA	142
	Definition	142
	Ætiology	143
	Symptoms :—	
	Prodromal	143
	Physical	143
	Mental	145
	Diagnosis	147
	Treatment	147
	Prognosis	148

		Page.
II.	Insanity of Myxodema	149
	Ætiology	149
	Symptoms :—	
	Physical	149
	Mental	150
	Diagnosis	151
	Pathology	151
	Treatment	151
	Prognosis	152
III.	Delusional Insanity	152
	(Paranoia, Megalomania, Mania of pride and grandeur, &c., &c.)	
	Definition	153
	Ætiology	154
	Symptoms :—	154
	Physical	154
	Mental	155
	Diagnosis	158
	Treatment	158
	Prognosis	158
IV.	Chronic Metabolic Toxæmia	158
	Ætiology	159
	Symptoms :—	
	Physical	159
	Mental	159
	Diagnosis	160
	Treatment	160
	Prognosis	160

CHAPTER XII.

Insanities of Toxic Origin—(*contd.*)

GROUP II.

Insanities due to Bacterial Toxæmias.

I.	Excited Melancholia	161
	Ætiology	162

		Page.
	Symptoms:—	162
	Prodromal..	162
	Physical ..	163
	Mental ..	163
	Diagnosis ..	164
	Treatment ..	165
	Prognosis ..	165
II.	MANIACAL EXCITEMENT WITH CONFUSION (Mania)..	166
	ACUTE MANIA:—Ætiology ..	168
	Symptoms:—	
	Prodromal..	168
	Physical ..	169
	Mental ..	172
	Diagnosis ..	174
	Treatment ..	174
	Prognosis ..	175
	MANIA FOLLOWING ON THE PUERPERIUM ..	175

CHAPTER XIII.

INSANITIES OF TOXIC ORIGIN—(*contd.*)

GROUP II.

INSANITIES DUE TO BACTERIAL TOXÆMIAS—(*contd.*)

III.	FOLIE CIRCULAIRE:—	
	Definition ..	177
	Ætiology ..	177
(*a*)	Stage of Elevation ..	178
	Symptoms:—	
	Prodromal ..	178
	Physical ..	178
	Mental ..	179
	Diagnosis ..	180
	Treatment ..	181
	Prognosis ..	182

		Page.
(b)	Stage of Depression ..	182
	Symptoms :—	
	Physical ..	182
	Mental ..	182
	Diagnosis ..	183
	Treatment ..	183
	Prognosis ..	183
IV.	KATATONIA ..	184
	Definition ..	184
	Ætiology ..	184
	Symptoms ..	144
(a)	Prodromal ..	184
(b)	Acute Stage of Onset ..	185
	Physical ..	185
	Mental ..	186
	Diagnosis ..	186
	Treatment ..	186
	Prognosis ..	187
(c)	Stage of Stupor ..	187
	Physical ..	187
	Mental ..	188
	Diagnosis ..	189
	Treatment ..	189
	Prognosis ..	189
(d)	Stage of Excitement ..	189
	Physical ..	190
	Mental ..	190
	Diagnosis ..	190
	Treatment ..	191
	Prognosis ..	191
V.	HEBEPHRENIA ..	191
	Definition ..	192
	Ætiology ..	192
	Symptoms :—	
	Prodromal ..	193
	Physical ..	193
	Mental ..	194
	Diagnosis ..	195

	Page.
Treatment	196
Prognosis	196

CHAPTER XIV.

INSANITIES OF TOXIC ORIGIN—(*contd.*)

GROUP III.

INSANITIES DUE TO THE ABUSE OF DRUGS AND ALCOHOL.

I. INSANITY DUE TO THE ABUSE OF CANNABIS INDICA	197
(*a*) Ganjah	197
(*b*) Bhang	198
(*c*) Charas	198
(*d*) Haschisch	198
Ætiology	198
Symptoms	200
(*a*) Acute Cases:—	
1. Acute Intoxication	201
Symptoms :—	
Physical	201
Mental	201
Treatment	202
2. Transitory Excitement	202
Symptoms :—	
Physical	202
Mental	203
Diagnosis	203
Treatment	203
Prognosis	203
(*b*) Chronic cases :—	204
Symptoms	204
Prognosis	204
II. INSANITY DUE TO THE ABUSE OF ALCOHOL ..	204
Ætiology	206
Varieties	206
(*a*) Acute Intoxication	207

Page.

Symptoms:—
Physical 207
Mental 207
Treatment 207
(*b*) Delirium Tremens 208
Symptoms:—
Physical 208
Mental 208
Diagnosis 209
Treatment 209
Prognosis 210
(*c*) Mania à potu:—
Ætiology 210
Symptoms:—
Physical 210
Mental 211
Diagnosis 211
Treatment 211
Prognosis 212
(*d*) Chronic Alcoholic Insanity 212
Ætiology 212
Symptoms:—
Physical 212
Mental 214
Diagnosis 215
Treatment 216
Prognosis 217
(*e*) Dipsomania 217

CHAPTER XV.

Insanities of Toxic Origin—(*concld.*)

GROUP III.

Insanities due to the abuse of Drugs and Alcohol—(*contd.*)

III. Insanity due to the abuse of opium and morphia 219
Morphia 220

		Page.
	Symptoms :—	
	Physical	221
	Mental	222
	Diagnosis	223
	Treatment	223
	Prognosis	224
IV.	ABUSE OF COCAINE	224
	Symptoms :—	
	Physical	224
	Mental	224
	Diagnosis	225
	Treatment	225
	Prognosis	225
V.	ABUSE OF ETHER AND CHLOROFORM	225
VI.	PARALDEHYDE HABIT	225
VII.	MERCURIAL AND LEAD POISONING	226
VIII.	IODOFORM POISONING	226
IX.	CARBON BISULPHIDE POISONING	226
X.	THYROID POISONING	227

CHAPTER XVI.

NERVOUS DISEASES COMPLICATED BY MENTAL DERANGEMENTS.

I.	EPILEPSY	228
	Ætiology	232
	Symptoms :—	
	Physical	232
	Mental	234
	Insanity associated with epilepsy	236
(1)	Epileptic Idiocy	236-237
(2)	Pre-epileptic Insanity	236-237
(3)	Masked epilepsy	236-237
(4)	Post-epileptic psychoses	236-238
(5)	Chronic epileptic insanity	236-239
	Diagnosis	239

		Page.
	Treatment	240
	Prognosis	242

CHAPTER XVII.

Nervous Diseases complicated by Mental Derangements—(*contd.*)

II.	General Paralysis of the Insane	244
	Ætiology	246
	Symptoms :—	
(*a*)	Prodromal	247
	Physical	247
	Mental	247
(*b*)	First stage :—Physical	248
(*c*)	Second stage :—Physical	250
(*d*)	Third stage :—Physical	251
	Mental Symptoms :—	252
	First stage	252
	Second stage	253
	Third stage	254
	Diagnosis	254
	Treatment	254
	Prognosis	256

CHAPTER XVIII.

States of Mental Enfeeblement.

I.	Idiocy and Imbecility	257
	Ætiology	257
	Symptoms	260
	Physical	261
	Mental	264
	Types of Idiocy	267
	Treatment	274
II.	Dementia	279

		Page.
(a)	Secondary Dementia	280
	Ætiology	280
	Symptoms :—	
	Physical	281
	Mental	282
	Treatment	285
(b)	Organic Dementia	285
	Symptoms :—	
	Physical	287
	Mental	287
	Diagnosis	287
	Treatment	287
	Prognosis	288

CHAPTER XIX.

Psychoses associated with Physical Diseases.

I.	Phthisis and Insanity	289
	Mental Symptoms	290
	Diagnosis	291
	Treatment	291
	Prognosis	291
II.	Malaria and Insanity	291
III.	Sunstroke and Insanity	292
IV.	Influenza and Insanity	294
	Symptoms	295
	Treatment	296
	Prognosis	296
V.	Rheumatic Fever and Insanity	296
	Treatment	297
	Prognosis	298
VI.	Heart Disease and Insanity	298
	Prognosis	298
VII.	Syphilis and Insanity	298
	Savage's Scheme	299
	Treatment	302
	Prognosis	303

		Page.
VIII.	CHOREA AND INSANITY	303
	Ætiology	303
	Symptoms	303
1.	Choreic Mania	304
2.	Choreic Stupor	304
3.	Choreic Delusional Insanity	304
4.	Huntington's Chorea	304
	Treatment	305
	Prognosis	305
IX.	PREGNANCY AND INSANITY	306
X.	MENSTRUATION AND INSANITY	306

CHAPTER XX.

PHYSICAL CONDITIONS LIABLE TO COMPLICATE INSANITY.

I.	HÆMATOMA AURIS	308
	Symptoms	309
	Treatment	309
II.	LESIONS OF THE OSSEOUS SYSTEM	310
III.	WOUNDS, ULCERS, etc.	311
IV.	MICRO-ORGANISMAL DISEASES	312
	Phthisis	313
	Pneumonia	313
	Dysentery and Diarrhœa	814
	Malaria	315
V.	MENSTRUAL DERANGEMENTS	316

CHAPTER XXI.

GENERAL TREATMENT.

Recognition and Treatment of Prodromata ..	319
Prophylaxis	319
Training of children with neurotic heredity ..	321
Condition of alimentary tract	322
Artificial Feeding	322

		Page.
(*a*)	Œsophageal tube	322
(*b*)	Nasal tube	323
	Fever in the insane	324
	Hyperpyrexia	324
	Subnormal temperatures	325
	Convalescence	325
	Routine exercise and amusements	325
	Mechanical Restraint :—	
1.	Padded Room	326
2.	The Sheet	327
3.	The Straitwaistcoat	327
4.	The Gloves or Mittens	328
5.	Dr. Wolffe's "Protective Bed"	329
	Hypnotism and hypnotic suggestion	330
	Serumtherapy	331
	Drugs	331
	Sedatives and hypnotics	333
	Opium and Chloral	334
	Paraldehyde	334
	Hyoscine and hyoscyamine	335
	The Bromides	336
	Sulphonal, Trional and Veronal	336
	Isopral	337
	Thyroid Treatment	337

APPENDICES.

FORMS, ETC. .. .. 340—350

CHAPTER I.

THE MEDICO-LEGAL ASPECT OF INSANITY IN INDIA.

THE medico-legal responsibilities of the medical profession in connection with its dealings with insanity are heavy and varied.

In addition to our statutory duties, judges, lawyers, etc., constantly call for medical aid in the solution of various questions. Thus an extra responsibility is thrown on our shoulders besides those relating to the liberty of the subject, civil capacity and control of property.

Still again in private practice the medical practitioner is constantly met by most delicate questions, of a medico-social character, owing to the impossibility of finding elsewhere so qualified an adviser as the medical attendant.

All these duties undoubtedly call for much care, searching enquiry into facts and above all grave consideration, not only of these facts, but also of the probable results of any advice given or action taken.

DISPOSAL OF THE PATIENT.

Several trying questions arise here. *Can we undertake the responsibility of treating the case at his own home?*

Should he be prevented from transacting business?

Must he be placed under the care of attendants and a certain amount of restraint?

Are we justified in taking the gravest action of all and sending the patient to an asylum?

In doubtful cases, or in the early stages of the disease, these are undoubtedly serious steps to take and involve a heavy responsibility. The patient says he is quite well, resents greatly the slightest attempt to curtail his liberty and threatens all and sundry with the most dire consequences.

Under these circumstances the doctor should make it be clearly understood that he is simply and solely an adviser and will take no legal responsibility whatsoever for any action taken to control the patient. It is on the relatives, who have a legal right and moral duty as regards the patient, that this responsibility falls, not on the doctor whose sole legal power is to grant certificates.

In fact all steps taken in the treatment of the case, such as curtailment of liberty, removal to homes or asylums, etc., etc., should, in every case, be authorised by a relative, not necessarily the nearest relative, but any relative whether by blood, marriage or adoption. I would strongly advise family councils being held, whenever possible, under these circumstances, and, if husband or wife be the patient, endeavour to have representatives of both families present at the discussion.

It must be remembered also that, in treating cases in private houses, any attendants are technically and legally the servants of the relatives and under their orders, however much in fact they may be under the doctor's deputed authority.

In India a patient can be treated in his own home without certification as long as his friends desire and so long as he is under proper control and not badly treated. Illtreatment of an insane, besides being a reason for his confinement in an asylum, also renders those responsible for it liable to heavy punishment. (Sect. 15 (2), Act IV of 1912.)

ADMISSION INTO ASYLUMS.

1. **On a petition from the patient himself.**—Any person in charge of an asylum, with the consent of two of the visitors of the asylum, on a written application from the intending boarder, may receive and lodge as a boarder in such asylum any person who is desirous of submitting himself to treatment. (Sect. 4 (1), Act IV, 1912.)

2. **Reception Orders on petition of relatives or others.**—The husband or wife, or any other relative of the patient may submit an application for a reception order to the Magistrate within whose jurisdiction the lunatic ordinarily resides. If such petition be presented by any one else it must contain a statement as to why it is not submitted by a relative, of the connection of the petitioner with the alleged lunatic, and of the circumstances under which he presents the petition. No person can present a petition who has not attained the age of majority, as determined by the law to which he is subject, or who has not seen the patient

personally within fourteen days before the presentation of the petition.

The petition must be in the prescribed form (App. I. A. q. v.) and must be signed and verified by the petitioner, and the statement of prescribed particulars (App. I. B.) must be signed and verified by the person making such statement. It must be supported by two medical certificates in due order (App. II q. v.), on separate forms. One of these must be from a gazetted medical officer, or a medical practitioner declared by general or special order of the Local Government a medical officer for the purposes of this act. If either certificate be signed by any relative, partner or assistant of the lunatic or the petitioner, this fact should be noted in the petition, and, where the person signing is a relative, the exact degree of relationship should also be given. If any previous application has been made in any Court for an enquiry into the mental capacity of the alleged lunatic, this must also be noted and a certified copy of the order made thereon should be attached to the petition.

On receipt of the petition the Magistrate, if he considers there are grounds for proceeding further, must personally examine the alleged lunatic, unless for reasons, which he records in writing, he considers this inadvisable or inexpedient.

If satisfied he may at once grant a reception order (App. III q. v.) Failing this, he must fix a date (notification of which must be sent to the petitioner and to any others to whom notice should be given in the opinion of the Magistrate), for the consideration of the petition. The Magistrate may also pass such orders as he thinks fit for the suitable custody of the alleged lunatic pending the conclusion of the enquiry.

On considering the petition the Magistrate may make a reception order (App. III) or dismiss the petition, or adjourn the same for further evidence or enquiry. He may also make such orders as to payment of costs as he thinks fit.

If the petition be dismissed the Magistrate must record his reasons in writing and the petitioner must be furnished with a copy of the order.

No reception order can be made under petition, except in the case of a lunatic who is dangerous and unfit to be at large, unless the Magistrate is satisfied that the person in charge of an asylum is willing to receive the lunatic, or the petitioner or some other person gives an undertaking to pay for the maintenance of the lunatic.

3. **Reception Orders otherwise than by petition.**— *Any European subject to the terms of the Army Act and declared a lunatic,* under the military regulations in force at the time, may be removed to an asylum which has been duly authorised for the purpose by the Governor-General in Council, on a reception order (App. IV) signed by any administrative medical officer to whom such removal may seem necessary.

Every police officer in charge of a police station may arrest or cause to be arrested all *wandering or dangerous lunatics.* Such persons must be forthwith taken before a Magistrate. If the Magistrate thinks fit he shall cause such persons to be examined by a medical officer and make any further enquiries as seem necessary. If satisfied that such a person is a lunatic and on receipt of a proper medical certificate, the Magistrate then passes a reception order (App. V & VI) for the admission of such lunatic into an asylum, or licensed asylum, (App. V & VI) at the wish of relatives of the insane. If any friend or relative of the lunatic enters into a bond for the due care of the lunatic and the prevention of his injuring himself or others the Magistrate may, if he thinks fit, make him over to the care of such friend or relative without passing a reception order.

Every officer in charge of a police station must immediately report to the Magistrate *all cases of lunatics not properly cared for and controlled, or who he has reason to believe are cruelly treated.* The Magistrate then causes the lunatic to be brought before him and summons such relative or other person who ought to have charge of him. An order is then passed for the proper care and treatment of the lunatic, wilful neglect of which renders the transgressor liable to imprisonment for not more than one month. If, however, the Magistrate deems it advisable he may act as in the preceding paragraph, obtain a medical certificate and pass an order for the lunatic's reception in an asylum.

4. **Detention under Observation.**—A Magistrate may, by order in writing, authorise the detention of an alleged lunatic in suitable custody under medical observation for such period, not exceeding 10 days, as may seem to him necessary to determine the state of the person's mind. Such period may be extended from time to time by further orders for periods not exceeding 10 days, if

such extensions seem necessary to the Magistrate. In any case no person can be detained for any period longer than 30 days.

In Presidency-towns or Rangoon the Commissioner of Police has magisterial powers in the above respects, and any officer of the police force not below the rank of an Inspector, has the powers of an officer in charge of a police-station.

Detention pending removal to an Asylum.—When a reception order has been passed, the Magistrate, for reasons which he must record in writing, may direct that the lunatic may be detained in suitable custody pending his removal to an asylum.

RECEPTION AFTER INQUISITION.

A lunatic, so found by inquisition, may, in the case of those subject to the jurisdiction of the High Courts of Fort William, Madras and Bombay, be admitted into an asylum on an order made by, or under, the High Courts (Chap. IV, Act IV, 1912). In the case of those subject to the jurisdiction of a District Court a similar order from the District Court is sufficient (Chap. V, Act IV, 1912). In such cases the Court passing the order must, on the application of the person in charge of the asylum, make an order for the payment of the cost of maintenance of the lunatic in the asylum and direct the recovery of such sums from the estate of the lunatic or of any person legally bound to maintain him. Where no adequate means of support exists, the Court certifies to the fact in lieu of passing the above order.

MEDICAL CERTIFICATES. (APPENDIX II).

Every certificate under this Act (Act IV, 1912), must be signed by a medical officer or practitioner, as the case may be, and must be in the prescribed form. It must contain a concise statement of the facts observed by the person certifying which lead him to the conclusion of insanity, and these facts should be clearly differentiated from those communicated to him by others. All such certificates are of the character of evidence and have the same weight as if verified on oath.

No reception order can be passed unless the person, or each person, certifying to insanity, has examined the alleged lunatic not more than seven clear days before the presentation of the petition, or, in all other cases, not more than seven clear days before the passing of the order. Where two certificates are required, those signing the certificates must examine the alleged lunatic separately from each other.

No Magistrate can make a reception order for the admission of any lunatic into any Government asylum outside the province in which he holds jurisdiction, unless by any general or special order of the Governor-General in Council.

DISCHARGE OF LUNATICS.

Discharge of Boarders admitted on a personal application.—A boarder received into an asylum on these terms cannot be detained for more than 24 hours after having given notice in writing, to the person in charge of the asylum, of his desire to leave such asylum.

Discharge of Non-Criminal Lunatics.—Three of the visitors of any asylum, one of whom must be a medical officer, may, by order in writing, direct the discharge of any person detained in such asylum. Notice of the discharge shall be immediately given to the authority under whose orders the lunatic was admitted.

Lunatics detained under a reception order made on a petition shall be discharged on the application in writing, to the person in charge of the lunatic asylum, of the person who submitted the petition, provided the lunatic is certified in writing as not dangerous nor unfit to be at large.

A person detained under the orders of a military administrative medical officer must be kept until his discharge under military regulations, or until the officer, making the order, applies for his transfer to the military authorities in view of his removal to England. Whenever such a person appears fit for discharge on account of recovery, or his discharge becomes necessary for some other reason, such person must be brought before the visitors of the asylum. On the visitors confirming the recommendation for discharge, the G. O. C., or other officer authorised to order the admission of such persons into an asylum, shall forthwith direct him to be discharged in accordance with the military regulations in force.

Discharge on undertaking of a relative.—Any relative or friend of a lunatic may apply to the authority, who signed the reception order, for the release of the lunatic. A report is then called for from the Superintendent of the asylum and the visitors, or one of them who must be a medical man. If this report be satisfactory the committing authority, after obtaining a sufficient undertaking (App. VII & VIII), from the relative of the lunatic for his care and safe custody, may pass an order for him to be handed over to his relative.

Discharge of persons admitted on a Magistrate's order and subsequently found sane on an inquisition under Chap. IV or V, Act IV of 1912.—When this occurs the alleged lunatic must be at once discharged from the asylum, on the production of a certified copy of the finding.

TRANSFER OF LUNATICS.

A lunatic may be removed from one asylum to another in the same province at the orders of the Local Government, or to another asylum in any part of British India by order of the Governor-General in Council.

ESCAPE AND RECAPTURE.

Any lunatic escaping from an asylum may be recaptured and brought back by any police officer or by any officer or servant of the asylum. Except, however, in the case of criminal lunatics, or European lunatics subject to the provisions of the Army Act, this power does not extend beyond a month from the date of the escape.

ILLEGAL DETENTION.

Act IV of 1912, Sec. 93 further enacts that anyone who, otherwise than in accordance with this Act, receives or detains a lunatic or alleged lunatic in an asylum, or for gain detains two or more lunatics in any place not being an asylum, is liable to imprisonment for a term not exceeding two years, to a fine, or to both.

CERTIFICATION OF PATIENT.

The grounds for certifying a patient and sending him to an asylum are not solely danger, accruing to the patient or the public by his remaining at large, but firstly and mainly the due care and treatment of the case. This being so the medical man's first duty is to decide on the definite reasons for such a course. Having done this, he must then convince the patient's relatives of the necessity for certification. In doing this avoid pressing them at first if they seem disinclined or averse to take such action. Simply explain the reasons for the step, point out the risks, and that the responsibility lies on them and not on the doctor. There is always a chance that certification may be the cause of legal action, and, in some rare cases, it may be necessary before certification to get a letter from some responsible person protecting you from such risk. As a rule, however, no action can stand if there is no reasonable ground for imputing to the doctor want of good faith or reasonable care. In the case of beggars and others sent up for examination by the police, etc., the chief responsibility undoubtedly lies on the medical man to whom the question of asylum treatment is referred and on whose opinion the authorities are obliged to act.

In certification the first thing, of course, to decide is, "*Is the patient insane?*" Having decided this endeavour to find what form of insanity the patient labours under, making use of any signs of mental disease observed by yourself, and also any facts proving it told to you by others who have seen the patient.

Next arises the question "*Is the patient a proper person to be detained under care and treatment?*" The chief grounds for this are, (*a*) danger to himself or others, (*b*) disturbance of the public peace, (*c*) inability to care for, or manage himself and his affairs, (*d*) acute mental symptoms of any kind, (*e*) amenability to curative treatment which cannot be applied without certification. Various questions—social, monetary and domestic—have to be determined here. One has to decide the reasons for his removal from home, how he will regard it after his recovery, how it will affect his business and, last and not least, what legal risk there is to oneself and his relations. If you cannot decide all these in one interview with the patient, see him, if necessary, several times, and make sure of your facts and reason in every way. Having done so then complete the first and legal part of the form with as much care as if you were answering an important question in an examination.

Then comes the "*facts indicating insanity observed by myself.*" Think of what the patient says and how he says it, of what he does and how he does it and of what he looks like. Put in first the most evident and indisputable insane delusions the patient labours under, as crisply and concisely as you can. Next note mutism, incoherence of speech, shouting, outrageous conduct, loss of memory, volition or reasoning power. Wherever possible quote verbatim from the patient some phrase or remark of convincing proof. In noting delusions it is at times necessary to note "which is a delusion" after them, thus "says he owns 10 lakhs of rupees" might possibly be true and would require to be noted, but "says he is Allah!" requires no remark. Note next the patient's appearance, expression and manner and, if you have known him before, note any changes from his normal condition. Avoid giving facts that do not indicate insanity, but in some cases, where such clear evidence as above is not available, lesser things put in a cumulative way might suffice us. Thus "his manner is listless and his looks vacant. Speech incoherent and irrelevant. Takes no interest in any thing. His whole appearance gives the impression of one unfit to manage his affairs" will quite suffice even when unsupported by "*Facts indicating insanity communicated to me by others*," which are important as subsidiary but not essential points of the certificates. Here insert descriptions of aggravations of conduct and speech, of attempts at or threats of suicide or homicide, etc., and in every case note down the name of the informant. Having completed this sign your name at the foot and then go carefully over the whole document and ensure its accuracy.

Immense tact is often required to bring out the real condition of the patent's mind even when one knows on good evidence that he is insane, and still more so is this the case when he knows or thinks you are a doctor come to certify him. In all cases find out all you can about a patient beforehand and especially regarding hallucinations or delusions if such exist, but even then in some cases you will find it hard, in fact impossible, to get sufficient evidence for certification even though you know the man to be a dangerous lunatic.

Very rarely it happens that **certificates of sanity** are required from the medical man. These require the utmost care and circumspection and very careful enquiry into the facts of the man's life and behaviour. I have myself known a patient leave an asylum and return some hours later with a certificate of sanity signed by some thoughtless doctor. The patient considered it a huge joke, but the doctor would have found himself in an awkward predicament if, after obtaining his certificate, the patient had killed himself or some other person. Such certificates are required to set aside an order for a committee of the person and estate (Chaps. IV & V, Act IV, 1912), and sometimes before a man can resume employment or public appointments. On discharge from an asylum in whatever condition, a discharge certificate should be always sent to the magistrate of the place to which the patient belongs stating the fact of his discharge whether on security or not and his condition, *i.e.*, "cured," "improved," "unimproved."

THE TRANSFER OF LUNATICS TO ENGLAND.

This is often a matter of difficulty and raises various questions which the relatives of the patient invariably look for the medical man to solve.

As a rule, if the patient be a Government servant, or one of his family, domiciled in Great Britain, or able to pay for his maintenance there, or with relatives able and willing to pay the said maintenance, Government will arrange for his passage by troopship. In such cases an application should be submitted through the Local Government, stating the circumstances fully and accompanied by a medical officer's statement of the case. Occasionally a passage may be arranged for in this way for private individuals. Such cases are rare, however, and exceptional circumstances must be present before this can be done.

Where private individuals are concerned, the only chance generally is to obtain a passage on one or other of the smaller boats in the "off-season." To do this it is necessary to write to the various steamer companies, explaining the case fully and asking if they can arrange a passage. Many of the larger lines absolutely refuse such passengers and the greatest hope lies in smaller lines, like the B. I. S. N. Co., sailing from Calcutta in the hot weather. In these circumstances too the same conditions apply, and unless the patient be domiciled in Great Britain, or ample means of support can be obtained, he should not be sent to England. In all such cases a relative, whenever possible, and attendant, or attendants, should accompany the patient. It is as well to give carefully detailed written instructions to the person in charge of the patient before his departure, for these smaller boats carry no doctor as a rule and it is as well those in charge of the case should know how to act in case of emergency. For a similar reason it is as well to provide a supply of drugs, likely to be required on the voyage, with written instructions regarding each.

No medical certificate of insanity should ever be sent with such cases. A written statement of the case should go in all cases, but a medical certificate is useless in England, or indeed anywhere, once the patient has left India. On arrival at the end of the voyage the patient has to be seen and certified by two registered medical practitioners, and a proper reception order obtained from a sheriff or magistrate, before admission can be obtained into any asylum. In violent cases it is as well to arrange beforehand with some institution for the reception of such cases. The patient is then met on arrival by some of the staff, who see to all legal proceedings and save the relatives much trouble and worry.

MANAGEMENT OF PROPERTY.

Chaps. IV & V of Act IV of 1912, lay down the legal proceedings to be followed out in the disposal of a lunatic and his estate. Chap. IV applies to those liable to the jurisdiction of the Supreme Courts and lays down that on the application of any person related, by blood or marriage, to the alleged lunatic, or on application by the Advocate-General, an enquiry may be ordered by the Court as to whether the alleged lunatic is of unsound mind and incapable of managing his affairs, also regarding his property, next of kin and such other matters as may appear necessary to the Court. Such enquiry may be held by the Court itself, by any Judge of the Court or by any principal Court of original jurisdiction in civil cases within whose jurisdiction the alleged lunatic may be. The Court may require the alleged lunatic to attend at any place within 20 miles of his residence for the purposes of examination, or may authorise any person or persons to have access to the said lunatic for purposes of examination; except that where the person is a female such order will be regulated by the rules in force for the examination of such persons in other cases. The Court has power to amend the original report or to order a new enquiry if it appear necessary, and may also make orders respecting the costs of the enquiry. After the enquiry, if necessary, a committee of the person and estate of the lunatic is appointed by the Court, and the Court by such order of appointment, or by subsequent order, grants such powers to the committee as shall be deemed necessary and proper, except that such powers shall not extend to the sale or mortgage of any part of the estate, or to the lease of any immovable property for terms exceeding three years. The Master of the Court has power to make enquiries regarding the management of the estate and can determine how many and which of the relatives of the lunatic shall attend such enquiry. The Court, on receipt of the Master's report, has power to pass such orders regarding the management, sale or mortgage of the estate as may be deemed necessary, the committee having power to execute all such deeds and conveyances as may be necessary for the carrying out of such orders. If the lunatic be a partner of a firm, the Court may order a dissolution of the partnership, and the committee carries this out in conjunction with the other members of the firm. Similarly the Court may order the disposal of a business, of a lease or underlease, or may assume charge of a lunatic's landed property with a view to the proper management of the same. The Court can also apply property for the maintenance of the lunatic and his family, without appointing a committee, if it be found necessary that this be done in an inexpensive manner, or in cases where the lunacy is reported as of a temporary character. The Court has also power to order a second enquiry if it be reported that the lunacy has ceased, and, if such be found to be the case, may then pass an order rescinding all past orders on such conditions as shall seem proper.

Chap. V applies to persons not subject to the jurisdiction of the Supreme Court and delegates the powers of enquiry, etc., to the Civil Court within whose judicature the lunatic resides. The application in this case may be made by any relative of the alleged lunatic, or by any public curator appointed under Act XIX of 1841, by the Government pleader or by the Collector on behalf of the Court of Wards. Similar powers of enquiry are granted here as in Chap. IV to the Supreme Court, and if the lunatic reside more than fifty miles from where the Court is held the enquiry may be delegated to any subordinate Court. The appointment of guardians of person and estate is practically the same as under Chap. IV, except that all proceedings in regard to the estate are subject to the control of the District Court or the Collector. The management of the estate also is to all intents and purposes similar to that laid down in Chap. IV, but, in addition, an inventory of the estate has to be submitted within six months, and an annual account of its management rendered within 3 months of the close of the year of the era current in the district. If the accuracy of such inventory or accounts be impugned, the Court may enquire summarily into the matter, or refer such petition to any subordinate Court or the Collector. Power is given to remove any manager, for sufficient cause, and order him to furnish accounts and hand over the estate to any other person appointed by the Court. In the event of the manager refusing to do this, or to furnish the inventory or the annual accounts mentioned above, the Court has power to impose a fine not exceeding Rs. 500. Power is given in certain cases for the Court to apply the estate for the maintenance of the lunatic and his family without the appointment of a manager, as under Chap. IV, and also to institute a second enquiry when the lunatic is alleged to have recovered.

CRIMINAL RESPONSIBILITY.

Medical men are often called on to give evidence as to the presence or not of mental disease in persons accused of crime to enable the law to fix or to absolve from responsibility. The forms of insanity mainly related to crime are mania, epileptic insanity, delusional insanity, alcoholic insanity, sometimes puerperal insanity, acute melancholia, sometimes dementia and amentia, also the so-called "Impulsive Insanities," *i.e.*, kleptomania, pyromania, etc., which are very frequently seen in women about the time of a menstrual period. Some of these cases when complicated with the effects of drunkenness are often most puzzling, both to medical men and lawyers, when crime has resulted. As a rule, however, and I think this is the experience of most alienists, crimes are usually committed in the incipient stages of insanity, the reason probably being that the more advanced cases have been placed under proper control and supervision, and it is they, who have not yet given grounds for being restrained and who are uncontrolled, who suddenly lose their senses or are seized by a sudden impulse and commit a crime, there being no restraining hand to withhold them. Drunkenness is not held to excuse but rather aggravate crime, though alcoholic insanity exempts from punishment. I think the latest accepted code of responsibility may be taken as that propounded by Mr. Justice Stephen and quoted by Dr. Clouston in his book from which much of the material for this section has been taken. He says: "The proposition which I have to maintain and explain is, that if it is not, it ought to be, the law of England that no act is a crime if the person who does it is, at the time when it is done, prevented, either by defective mental power or by any disease affecting his mind, from controlling his own conduct, unless the absence of the power to control has been produced by his own default."

There are undoubtedly many cases most difficult to decide—cases just on the borderland, cases of vice and mental disease most puzzlingly intermingled, cases of drink taken when the consequences were well known and resulting in brutal crime, the result of the mad frenzy caused by the excess. In all cases one must go into the case absolutely unprejudiced in every way, enquire carefully about the man's antecedents, his habits, whether he has ever had fits, etc., etc., and, especially where the crime is of a specially revolting character or done without any apparent motive, great care should be taken in looking for epilepsie larvée in the former and delusions of persecution or signs of paranoia in the latter case.

When *giving your evidence* be concise and clear, remember you are talking to non-medical men and avoid abstruse medical phrases as far as possible, and if you have to use one, be ready with an explanation of it. Avoid theories and quoting authorities as much as ever you can, but state facts and the conclusions you yourself come to from these and be prepared to justify these if necessary. It must be remembered too that we are seldom conversant with the whole facts on both sides, and we are often regarded and treated as partisans. Under present conditions this is unavoidable, however derogatory and galling it may be, and one must just be prepared for the inevitable cross-examination. During this keep cool, answer as concisely as possible, avoid being drawn into lengthy discussions and generalities, but stick to your facts and, if necessary, insist on answering a double barrelled question by "Yes and No." Don't mind saying "I don't know" and you will come out all right.

CRIMINAL LUNATICS.

In Indian asylums the so-called *Criminal Lunatics* are divided into 3 classes :—

A. Those unable to stand their trial owing to their mental condition rendering them unfit to make their defence (Seçt. 466, Act V of 1898).

B. Those who have stood their trial and been found to have committed the crime while labouring under mental disease (Sect. 471, Act V of 1898).

C. Those who have been tried and sentenced, and, while undergoing their term of imprisonment, have become mentally affected and had to be sent to the asylum (Sect. 30, Act III of 1900).

Class A are detained as a rule until fit to make their defence ; they are then put on trial and as a rule returned to the asylum under class B. Under this class are included persons who, though not technically insane, are, through the loss of some special sense, such as being deaf and dumb, deprived of the power to make their defence. It seems hard on such cases, but, until some special legislation is brought in, it is hard to know what to do with them and it will be difficult to legislate with due justice both to such cases and the community at large.

Class B, as a rule, have to spend at least 3 years in an asylum without showing any signs of insanity and are thereafter sent, as a rule, to gaol for a further probation of 3 years. The times vary, however, according to the cause of the disease, etc.

Class C, if sane on the expiry of their sentence, are discharged as cured to their homes; otherwise they are transferred from the criminal to the non-criminal sections and treated as ordinary lunatics.

FEIGNED INSANITY.

The detection of this is one of the duties which at times fall to our lot and a very difficult one it is. Our chief aid lies in the fact that those feigning insanity, as a rule, know little if anything about it and overact their part. They mix up incoherent maniacal symptoms with silliness, talk no sense at all and pretend to know nothing, to have forgotten everything.

There is no fixed rule for detecting malingerers, but one has just to proceed in a regular methodical manner. Note carefully the character and severity of the symptoms and whether they correspond with any ordinary known type of insanity. Watch the patient carefully and continuously, at times openly and then again with secrecy, so that he does not know that he is being watched, and you will find when he fancies he is unobserved the symptoms cease, for no sane man can for long imitate maniacal frenzy. In the same way a man feigning acute mania perspires freely and cannot possibly feign the dry harsh skin and lips, furred tongue, high temperature, the constant restlessness and sleeplessness usually associated with this condition. Sensibility to pain should be tested and the state of the reflexes carefully examined into. A battery is at times useful in detecting such cases, and I have known wonderful "recoveries" occur with the casual mention in the patient's hearing of the cautery "a good large iron about 4″ dia. and at white heat, I think, if no improvement occurs by this evening." One is also often able to catch a malingerer by making a suggestion of some symptom "wanting in his case," and the chances are that by your next visit the "symptom" is much in evidence and this is specially so in feigned epilepsy. In certain types of insanity too a leucocytic count is of great aid in distinguishing between a malingerer or a genuine case.

At times a man really insane assumes an exaggerated insanity to make his friends think that the asylum is doing him harm, and hypochondriacal cases at times assume a grotesque more or less voluntary imitation of insanity to prove to their friends how really ill they are, and in hysteria it is also common. The British soldier at times feigns insanity in order to be sent to the hills or invalided home, and the sepoy for very similar reasons does the same, while in those awaiting trial the motive is readily to be found.

It is a common practice among natives of India to try and avoid the results of business transactions, or of deeds which they may have signed, by afterwards feigning insanity, and a word of caution is here necessary to a young practitioner or he may find himself in a very awkward position. Never be satisfied with merely half-an-hour's or even an hour's talk with your patient at your own bungalow, unless you have a fair knowledge of him previously, but delay a few days, visit him at unexpected hours at his own house and find out, in an unobtrusive way, something about him and his affairs from others besides his own relatives. This may seem unnecessary, perhaps even lose a patient or two, but the avoidance of a very uncomfortable half hour or more in Court is well worth it.

TESTAMENTARY CAPACITY.

Unfortunately, as a rule, we are not consulted at the time the will is made, when the real capacity of the testator could be examined into, but are placed in the witness-box after he is dead with most imperfect and one-sided information to go on, and probably more often than not strong motives for those consulting us to prevent our getting at all the facts.

In regard to wills we have to take a larger and wider view of the disturbances of the mental functions of the brains than those comprised under technical insanity. The dotard, the man dazed and sodden with drink, the man racked with agonising pain, the man rendered mentally unresisting and facile from exhausting disease and the near approach of death, may all require to have their testamentary capacity tested. In such cases it is of the greatest necessity that an experienced medical man should examine impartially as to the testamentary capacity of the person, before large sums of money are irrevocably dealt with in a document that above all things requires sound judgment for its validity. An important point to remember on this matter is that a lesser amount of mental capacity is needed for making a valid will than for managing property, or even for enjoying freedom from restraint. Patients in asylums during remissions of their disease and with insane delusions that did not affect the provisions of the will have been held to have made good wills by the highest tribunals.

When consulted in a matter of this kind, one should insist on seeing the patient alone, or at any rate with no one but a nurse or the family solicitor present. The points then to be considered are—1. *Is the patient free from the influence of drink or drugs and in his usual state?*

2. *Does he know the nature of what he is about to do and realise the result of the document he is to sign?*

3. *Is he free of, and uninfluenced by, insane delusions in regard to any of its provisions and also uninfluenced by a morbidly enfeebled mind?*

4. *Is there abnormal facility of mind from bodily disease, intemperate habits, weakness or any other cause, or is there any undue influence exercised from without.*

5. *Make the testator then enumerate his possessions and also all his relatives and any others he may wish to leave legacies to.*

6. *Then make him go over the particulars of the will he proposes to make, asking reasons for any dis-*

position of property that seems unjust or out of the ordinary, or for any relatives being omitted.

7. *Find for how long he has had these intentions and if possible get independent testimony from others.*

8. *Ascertain if possible the nature of the mental disorder the patient is suffering from.*

Senile patients often are very emotional and readily weep or become irritated, and this often indicates a lack of mental power and volitional resistance. Persons suffering from apoplexy or paralysis may have very varying degrees of mental power, from an almost normal mentalisation up to one of complete fatuity and want of memory.

In examining such a case one must be absolutely impartial, avoid any suggestions or expressions of opinion as to provisions to be made, and above all avoid influencing the testator in his views as to the disposition of his property. Also the greatest care must be taken to avoid sanctioning a "*bad will,*" no matter how good its provisions may be and how much trouble and expense may be avoided by doing so, as such an act would be most improper and illegal.

CONFIDENTIAL FAMILY ADVICE.

This is at times asked from the medical man as to the *propriety of marriages* when one party has had insanity or comes of a neurotic stock, as to the upbringing, education, etc., of children of markedly neurotic taint, or the significance of sudden changes in character, gross immorality, etc. Personally

I always strongly advise people against marrying into a neurotic or insane stock in the same way as I always strongly discountenance marriage between first cousins. A neurotic man may marry a plump, phlegmatic woman and good stock may result, but even here the risks are great and still more so, if the case is reversed and the woman be neurotic, hysterical and of markedly insane heredity. This of course does not apply where a sporadic case of insanity has occurred in the family or some member has suffered from senile breakdown resembling insanity, but only to families of undoubted neurotic stock.

As to the *unbringing of children of markedly insane or neurotic stock*, this should be undoubtedly on strictly physiological lines. They should be brought up in the country, or the hills. Their diet should be mainly milk and cereals. They should have short school hours and be encouraged to enter into sport and games as far as possible. Their lives and time should be systematised and at puberty special attention should be paid to them, as their sexual instincts are very much in evidence and apt to take unnatural forms. As to their occupations, these should be free from much headwork or excitement and should not be sedentary. Fixed salaried appointments with regular hours and holidays are the places for them. As a rule, however, such children come to no good and it is from this neurotic stock that the dipsomaniac, the impulsive criminal arises and by whom by far the largest number of places in our asylums are filled.

CHAPTER II.

CAUSATION OF INSANITY.

THE idea, I think, most commonly accepted as to the cause of insanity is that it is due to an unstable brain readily thrown into disorder by physical causes, nervous shock or mental strain, and that this instability is transmitted from one generation to another. Thus when a man who has suffered monetary losses, or a mother who has lost her child, becomes insane, the condition is at once believed to be directly due to the mental effect of such losses, and when a parturient woman becomes mentally deranged, it is, to use Clouston's words, "due to the physical cataclysm, the pains of labour, the excitement mental and bodily, the exhaustion, the loss of blood, septicæmia, the sudden diversion of the stream of vital energy from the uterus to the mammæ, the reflex disturbances on an unstable brain from the reproductive organs, these acting together or separately." To cases where no such causes are ascribable the term "idiopathic" is applied, or, as in some cases occurring in adolescence, the cause is said to be "cerebral involution."

Other views, however, have been promulgated of late years and now the toxic theory of the causation of insanity is daily gaining ground and becoming wider spread. Seventeen years ago Macpherson wrote: "The toxic basis of all forms of insanity is a presumption for which there is fairly good foundation but no proof." Now Bruce, in his work which bids fair to start a new era in psychiatrical methods, brings forward what, to those who have studied bacteriology fairly deeply, must be at least most convincing presumptive evidence of the truth of this, though, as he himself says, "there is still no direct proof and never will be, because the only satisfactory and irrefutable proof would be the experimental production of morbid mental states by the use of toxines and that is impossible."

Macpherson divides his causes of toxæmia into :—

A. Autointoxication as the result of (*i*) Physiological instability ; (*ii*) Defective metabolism ; (*iii*) Defective gland secretion ; (*iv*) Autointoxication from the alimentary tract ; (*v*) Autointoxication from the liver and kidneys.

B. Intoxication from micro-organisms introduced into the system.

C. Voluntary Intoxication by alcohol and drugs.

Though each of these causes is sufficient in itself to produce an attack of insanity, as a rule in all cases there is a combination of several of these causes. Thus with defective gland secretion or autointoxication from the alimentary canal, though primarily perhaps these may be the sole causes, yet soon the liver and kidneys become affected by the action of the toxines on them during the act of excretion, and in the end we have the double action. In the same way it can be seen that with the intoxications produced by micro-organisms, alcohol or drugs, though the primary effects may be due to these alone there is sooner or later superadded one or more of the sub-divisions of class *A*, owing to the action of these primary toxines on the rest of the organs of the body as well as on the central nervous system.

The term used to identify class *B*, *i.e.*, "micro-organisms introduced into the system," is in the majority of cases incorrect; for, as a rule, in most cases due to this cause the micro-organisms are found to infest some part of the alimentary canal, and it is their toxic products alone which are found to gain entrance into the general system and cause the nervous symptoms. Very often these organisms are normally present in the human alimentary system and it is some impairment of the general vitality, some derangement of the glandular secretion or metabolism, which either may allow the micro-organisms to increase to a pathological extent or may fail to destroy the toxines they produce, as is done in the healthy body. Very rarely indeed are micro-organisms to be found in the blood of insanes and when found they are invariably of the streptococci or staphylococci group. That these invasions are not, as has been stated, terminal affections, has been proved by Dr. Bruce, as the agglutinines produced by the action of the toxines of these organisms have been found in the blood of insanes who were not in the typhoid state.

Whatever the exciting cause of insanity may be, undoubtedly the chief predisposing cause is an unstable mental heredity. The sane are as liable as the insane to the exciting causes of insanity, but what will in a man without hereditary predisposition produce little or no effect, in one with hereditary predisposition will suffice to produce a severe attack of mental disease.

Hereditary predisposition here has a wider application than to those born of insane parents only. It should be looked on as including such defects as extreme nervousness, eccentricity, alcoholism, hysteria, epilepsy, vagabondage, and any want of balance in the mental developement, *e.g.*, extreme brilliancy in one direction combined with deficiency in others.

In addition to this the truth of the old adage "mens sana in corpore sano" is constantly brought home to us in asylum practice where almost daily we see striking proofs of it. Thus the offspring of syphilitic, gouty, rheumatic and phthisical patients are infinitely more liable to suffer from mental disorders than those sprung from healthy stock.

Probably the working of heredity is twofold, the patient starting life with an unstable nervous system which is readily influenced by toxines, which, in their turn, more readily gain access to it owing to the inefficiency of the natural defences of the body against them.

Hereditary predisposition manifests itself in various ways. The patient may be born an imbecile or may retain his mental balance till old age sets in. In some cases 2 or 3 generations may escape and one can in no way be sure of the form of derangement transmitted. Epileptics may beget imbeciles, alcoholics may beget maniacs and maniacs beget epileptics, and one and all of these may beget offspring who pass through life without showing any sign whatever of mental derangement. The maternal heredity is said to have the greatest effect on the disposition of the offspring, but the paternal heredity too is undoubtedly a strong factor in such cases. Asylum statistics in India on this point are most vague, owing to the meagre information as a rule received with each patient, fully 50% coming in without any family history whatever. Of the remaining 50% about 20—25% are noted as due to hereditary causes.

Child marriages which are so common, especially in Hindu communities, are undoubtedly a factor to be reckoned with in the ætiology of mental diseases. In such cases where one or both parties to the union has not arrived at maturity, setting aside for the moment the disastrous results to the offspring, the nervous and physical strain of such premature unions is bound to be enormous and tell heavily on the individual in later life. The offspring too in such cases are bound to be affected, at first by the immaturity of the parents and later by the vitality of the parents, lowered as it is by such premature sexual indulgence, and, as a result, the children of such marriages are very commonly rickety or tubercular, or show some of the other physical or nervous stigmata of degeneration, and it is among them that a very large proportion of cases of katatonia, hebephrenia and paranoia occur.

Consanguineous marriages and the greater stress of modern civilised life are at times brought forward as predisposing factors in the production of mental disease. The former can only influence it as tending to intensify a bad heredity, and the latter is a very questionable item, for the probability is that the stress and rush of life was just as great to our forbears in the past as it now seems to us when we arrive at the time for fending for ourselves. In fact, the only way by which modern life is likely to have effect, is that the tendency nowadays is to crowd together and live in large centres and under unnatural conditions which tend to lower vitality and weaken resistance to bacterial invasion.

In addition to the above, anything which impairs the general vitality and weakens resistance to bacterial invasion may be called a predisposing cause of insanity, *e.g.*, worry, great mental strain, exhausting and debilitating illnesses, sexual and alcoholic excesses, the "critical periods of life," *i.e.*, adolescence, the climacteric and puerperal states and senility, faulty sanitation, abuse of drugs such as opium and cocaine, shock and cerebral trauma, etc. Faulty upbringing and lack of moral training are also two most common and potent factors in the production of mental disease, causing as they do a deficiency in the developement of volition and self-control.

Exciting causes of Insanity.—Among male admissions into asylums in India undoubtedly the most common exciting cause is the abuse of drugs, especially of one form or another of *cannabis indica,* rather more than 25% of the total male admissions of whom a history can be obtained being admitted for this cause alone. Practically no females are admitted owing to this cause, the most common causes among them being fever, lactation and childbirth.

As already stated, the most prevalent view held at present is that the disease originates *de novo* in the deranged cells and fibres of the cortex of the brain, and that the physical symptoms concurrent with such disease are directly the result of the pathological changes in the cerebral cortex. This on a little consideration will, I think, be admitted by all to be rather too sweeping a statement, as it palpably assumes that the brain is immune from the results of disease affecting the body as a whole, takes no note of the physical symptoms which in the majority of cases precede insanity, and ignores altogether the fact that, in practically all cases, physical improvement precedes any change for the better in the mental condition.

With the theory of the toxic origin of insanity no such fault can be found. Its very essence is that a physical cause in all cases must precede the mental symptoms and, therefore, that a physical improvement must take place before any hope of improvement in the mental condition can be held. Bruce's work in this line also furnishes invaluable evidence in its favour, proving, as it does in certain cases, the presence of distinct hyperleucocytosis along with the presence of bacterial agglutinines in the blood. Still further we have in many cases changes in the integument and kidneys which indicate that the excretory system is straining its utmost to remove some deleterious substances from the organism.

At times the mental condition seems more of a functional nature, depending possibly on the diurnal rise and fall of the blood-pressure, or even varying to a still greater extent and depending on the 4 weekly curve hereafter noted as being present normally. In connection with this it is interesting to remember the derivation of the term "lunatic" which arose from an old-time belief that the phases of the moon were in some mysterious way connected with the course of insanity, this regular periodicity being readily explained, however, by the regular periodic rise and fall of the blood-pressure, the exacerbations of insanity as a rule occurring at its maxima or minima.

The exciting causes of insanity may be divided into two broad classes, (*a*) the *non-toxic,* and (*b*) the *toxic.*

(*a*) The chief **non-toxic cause** is probably exhaustion, either as the result of severe physical or mental effort, or severe illness, for when vitality is at a low ebb it is but natural that the brain should be affected both structurally and functionally as well as the other organs of the body, and the greater the hereditary predisposition of the patient the more readily will mental symptoms develope.

The other most common non-toxic causes of brain disease are probably brain injuries, and the results of hæmorrhage and traumatism. Other causes, as anæmia, cardiac disease and narrowing of the lumen of the blood-vessels are noted by some authors, but it seems to me incorrect to enter these here, as in all of them there is not only a possibility but a very great probability of intoxication; in anæmia an autointoxication probably from the intestinal tract and defective metabolism, and in the others an intoxication due to the cause of the cardiac and arterial conditions. Sudden deprivation of the special senses of sight and hearing occasionally brings on attacks of insanity.

(*b*) **Toxic causes.**—These may be divided into three groups :—

1. *Toxines of metabolic origin.* With these as a rule there are symptoms of severe nutritional disorder with diminished excretion from the skin, intestines and kidneys.

2. *Toxines of bacterial origin.* In these cases there is hyperleucocytosis, and agglutinines and alexines are present in the serum. Besides these there is a diminution in the amount of chlorides excreted in the urine, and at times boils, pustules and irritative rashes are seen on the skin. The organisms producing these conditions are, more often than not, normal inhabitants of the body which become able to produce their effect through a weakening of the natural defences of the body against bacterial infection, and these, as already noted, are specially prone to break down in those of marked neurotic heredity.

It is supposed by many that the bacteria normally present in the intestinal tract are there for some purpose and are essential for the due carrying on of certain physiological processes. Bruce in his work states that it is possible that their toxines act as a nervous stimulant, as he has noted in persons, who though not insane are extremely nervous and excitable, that the blood serum often contains agglutinines and alexines to such organisms as the staphylococci, etc., and cites cases of mental confusion and excitement seen by him, indistinguishable from acute mania, arising as the result of acute poisoning from the staphylococcus pyogenes aureus, the streptococcus pyogenes and the diplococcus pneumoniæ.

3. *Drug Toxæmia* includes poisoning by the various forms of cannabis indica, opium and morphia, cocaine, chloral and alcohol.

More often than not the mental condition is due to a combination of these causes, an exhaustion condition combining later in the progress of the disease with a toxæmic, or metabolic and bacterial toxæmias may be combined and produce mixed symptoms, and almost invariably alcoholic and similar drug toxæmias are combined both with metabolic and bacterial ones. It must also further be noted that the differences in working between two normal brains are still further exaggerated in disease, and that no two brains therefore can be expected to react in exactly the same manner even to the same toxæmia. The effects of brain habits must be remembered also as affecting sleep and the general routine life of the patient, for bad "brain habits" are much more easily acquired than good ones.

CHAPTER III.

CLASSIFICATION OF INSANITY.

MANY and varied are the classifications which have been put forward from time to time, some on a symptomatological, others on a clinical basis. They are all now, I think, generally regarded as inaccurate, unscientific and confusing; the former because they are based mainly on mental symptoms alone the physical symptoms being practically ignored, and the latter because at times predisposing causes or even symptoms have been mistaken for exciting causes. For these reasons I propose to place before my readers the tentative classification promulgated by Dr. Bruce, not as a final or complete one, but as a working basis. In it while still retaining some of the old nomenclature he has regrouped the affections broadly into insanities of non-toxic origin and insanities of toxic origin. It is undoubtedly on these lines that all future classification will be based, and moreover, such a classification, besides being simple and accurate, is a great help in deciding one as to the lines on which treatment of individual cases should be carried out.

BRUCE'S CLASSIFICATION.

I. INSANITIES OF NON-TOXIC ORIGIN.

1. *Exhaustion Insanity.*—A collection of physical and mental symptoms which are fairly constant and

occur as the result of some physical or mental strain, as the sequelæ of exhausting diseases such as typhoid, influenza, phthisis, etc., and most typically seen as the result of prolonged lactation.

2. *Insanity resulting from brain anæmia.*

3. *Insanity the result of gross brain lesion or traumatism.*

4. *Insanity resulting from deprivation of the special senses, particularly sight and hearing.*

II. Insanities of toxic origin.

Group A.—**Insanities the result of toxines of metabolic origin.**

1. *Acute Melancholia.*—A mental disease in which there is always depression, confusion and vivid hallucinations, associated with physical symptoms of malnutrition, and evidences of deficient excretion of the waste products of the body. The acute stage is of short duration, and is followed by recovery, or more commonly by a sub-acute stage of indefinite duration, in which the patient is always depressed, but may present a variety of mental symptoms, and in which the malnutrition persists together with deficient excretion of the waste products of the body. Hyperleucocytosis is never present.

2. *Insanity associated with deficient, excessive or altered secretion of the thyroid gland.*

3. *A variety of puerperal insanity.*

4. *Delusional Insanity.*—A definite disease process which in its later stages is characterized by fixed delusions, but whose early symptoms are very similar

to those of acute melancholia. The disease is at present described as progressive systematised insanity, mania of persecution and grandeur, megalomania and paranoia.

5. *Chronic Metabolic Toxœmia* (premature senility, chronic brain atrophy).

Group B.—**Insanities in which there is evidence of bacterial toxines being present in the blood, in which there is always a hyperleucocytosis, and in which bacterial agglutinines are frequently present in the serum.**

1. *Excited Melancholia.*—A mental disease in which there is depression, with constant noise and restlessness, but without marked mental confusion, with the symptom of hyperleucocytosis always present. Partial recoveries followed by exacerbations are very common, and the disease, if not recovered from, may terminate in a state of fixed delusion associated with chronic malnutrition. The condition rarely passes on to typical dementia.

2. *Maniacal Excitement with confusion* (Acute Mania).—A type of mental disease very variable in the intensity of the mental symptoms, but nearly always associated with maniacal excitement and confusion, with the symptom of hyperleucocytosis always present and generally persistent even after recovery. The disease may be continuous or recurrent, and may occur at any period of life. Complete or partial recovery is common, generally within three months from the onset of the symptoms, but one attack always predisposes to a second. Cases which do not recover generally become delusional, chronically noisy, restless and des-

tructive, and tend to terminate sooner or later in dementia. This disease is never associated with alternate periods of excitement and depression, although a condition of exhaustive stupor with confusion may follow the maniacal attack.

3. *Folie Circulaire.*—Mental elevation or depression without confusion—Kraepelin's manio-depressive insanity—which probably includes the simple mania and melancholia of most authors. A mental disease in which there may be either recurrent attacks of states of depression or states of elevation, or the states of depression and elevation may regularly alternate. In neither state is there typical mental confusion. The symptom of hyperleucocytosis is always present during the stage of elevation, but disappears on recovery. The stage of depression is frequently associated with a hyperleucocytosis, which is most marked in the cases in which there are alternate attacks of elevation and depression. The disease is apt to recur, attack following attack, but rarely, if ever, terminates in dementia.

4. *Katatonia.*—A disease which most frequently occurs in adolescence, and is characterised by a stage of acute onset in which fear, impulsive actions, confusion and vivid hallucinations are the chief mental symptoms. Hyperleucocytosis is always present, and in many cases the voluntary muscles are thrown into a state of rigidity or spasm of very variable duration.

The acute stage is followed by a stage of stupor without loss of consciousness, and the onset of stupor is associated with a very marked hyperleucocytosis. The voluntary muscles pass into a stage of resistiveness to passive movements, and in many cases efforts at voluntary movements are difficult, awkward or even impossible owing to counterstimuli or irritability of the opposing muscles. The stage of stupor may terminate in recovery or dementia, or the patient may pass into a stage of excitement, and then recover or become hopelessly demented. Until the disease terminates in dementia or recovery, the hyperleucocytosis is always more or less persistent. If the patient relapses, the disease may again pass through all the stages, but not infrequently patients, who have suffered from one attack of katatonia and recovered, if they relapse, present mental symptoms of excitement which, without a history of the first attack, are confusing and difficult to diagnose.

5. *Hebephrenia.*—A disease which occurs during adolescence, and is characterised on the physical side by delayed or arrested developement, by recurrent attacks of hyperleucocytosis and alterations in the pulse and temperature, and, on the mental side, by steadily progressive enfeeblement, incapacity for occupation, and occasional outbursts of excitement. In 80 per cent. of the cases affected the termination is hopeless dementia.

6. *Insanity after specific fevers.*—Where a deranged mental condition is met with after ordinary malaria, typhoid and other specific diseases of bacterial or micro-organismal origin.

Group C.—**Insanities the result of alcoholic and drug toxines.**

1. *Delirium tremens.*

2. *Alcoholic mania.*
3. *Chronic alcoholic insanity.*
4. *Morphinism.*
5. *Cocainism.*
6. *Chronic poisoning by alcohol, ether, chloroform, mercury, iodoform, lead, carbon bisulphide, paraldehyde, Indian hemp and thyroid.*

III. Nervous Diseases frequently complicated by Mental Diseases.

1. *Epilepsy.*
2. *General paralysis.*
3. *Dipsomania.*

IV. States of mental enfeeblement.

1. *Idiocy and imbecility.*
2. *The higher imbeciles.*
3. *Secondary dementia.*
4. *Organic dementia.*

CHAPTER IV.

DERANGEMENTS OF MENTALISATION.

The three most common conditions met with in asylums, in fact one might almost say the three, for all cases can be roughly grouped under one or other head, are those of morbid depression, of excitement and of elevation. These, though in all cases due primarily to some central disturbance, some disorder of the brain cortex, are frequently aggravated by derangements of the special sense centres, such as hallucinations, and most usually the centres of sight and hearing are those thus implicated.

Elevation and excitement are as a rule used as synonymous terms when maniacal conditions are being described, but this is incorrect and should be avoided whenever possible. True *elevation* or *exaltation* of spirits is only seen in cases, such as the exalted stage of folie circulaire, where there is complete absence of confusion, and it is generally associated with a feeling of intense happiness and well-being. *Excitement* on the contrary is as a rule associated with more or less mental confusion, and is seen usually at the onset of an attack of any of the acute insanities and most typically in acute mania.

Mental Confusion is a condition met with in varying degree in many types of insanity, from an inability to understand and answer simple questions to a state-of absolute fatuity where all power to grasp one's position and surroundings is lost. Some authors ascribe all conditions of confusion to toxæmias, but this is too sweeping a statement, for in mental exhaustion there is usually a condition of mild confusion in which no element of toxæmia can be found. On the other hand, in the elevation of folie circulaire, where there is indubitable evidence of toxæmia, there is complete absence of confusion, so the two conditions are in no way necessarily connected. Mental confusion is best seen in acute melancholia, acute mania, katatonia and toxæmias causing continued excitement.

Hallucinations are false sense impressions occurring without normal stimuli. Thus a patient may in the silence of the night imagine he hears voices abusing and threatening him when there is really not a sound to be heard, or he may imagine he is visited by friends who may be dead or miles away from him, and no one is really present by him. They may be due to either peripheral or central causes and are commonly associated with conditions of nervous exhaustion, or toxæmias.

Often for some time before the final breakdown the patient suffers from "noises in the head" and so on, and recognises these as false impressions, and it is only when this power to distinguish between true and false impressions is lost that the term hallucination is applicable. In such cases it is probable that the repeated hallucinations may be the cause of the insanity, for, as the brain is dependent on the reception of external sensory impressions for its normal working, the constant reception of such false impressions is bound to affect it.

Patients frequently deny the presence of hallucinations even when questioned with the utmost tact; as a rule, however, close watching will reveal them. Thus the patient in the middle of a conversation suddenly turns round and calls out "What?" or shouts out some reply to a question which he alone has heard, or he may assume a position of attentive listening when left alone, or carry on a conversation of which the on-looker can only hear the patient's remarks, though apparently the patient is quite able to hear the replies.

Aural Hallucinations are undoubtedly the most common and like all hallucinations tend to be most pronounced at night. They vary from simple rustlings, creakings and ringings of bells up to complete sentences. The symptoms of patients suffering from these vary from sitting in a position of strained attention with eyes fixed in the direction the sound is apparently coming from, to carrying on conversations with invisible persons or launching into volleys of apparently causeless abuse.

Visual Hallucinations are frequently associated with those of hearing, and are specially characteristic of alcoholic insanity or acute insanity complicated by alcoholic excess.

Hallucinations of taste and smell are commonly associated and as a rule are due to disordered alimentation. They are not commonly seen except in alcoholic cases, though hallucinations of smell are seen in women, associated with uterine and ovarian disease, and in men in association with the habit of self-abuse.

Hallucinations of sensation are most generally seen in delusional insanity and those cases associated with drugs, such as morphia and cocaine. They vary from mere tingling sensations to systematised hallucinations of persecution by electricity, of being run over by insects and all sorts of elaborate tortures. Such cases require careful watching as they are very frequently either homicidal or suicidal, their motive being revenge in the former case and in the latter escape from their imaginary enemies.

Illusions are sense impressions wrongly interpreted by the patient, *e.g.*, the patient may mistake the doctor for the king, or a dog for a tiger. They are very commonly seen in delirium tremens.

Insane Delusions are defined by Clouston as "a belief in something which would be incredible to people of the same class, education or race as the person who expresses it, the belief persisting in spite of proof to the contrary, this resulting from diseased working of the brain convolutions." The majority of delusions are as a rule the result of sensory hallucinations and so may be described as secondary, but some, especially in states of depression, are primary and directly due to the intense feeling of misery.

Delusions are divided into two divisions, permanent or fixed delusions, and temporary or transitory delusions. These again are subdivided into delusions of suspicion or persecution, and delusions of pride or grandeur, the former being typically seen in paranoia.

and alcoholic insanity, the latter in general paralysis of the insane.

Stupor is defined by Clouston as "a morbid condition in which there is mental and nervous lethargy and torpor, in which impressions on the senses produce little or no outward effect, in which the faculty of attention is, or seems to be, paralysed, in which there is no sign of originating mental power, in which the higher reflex functions of the brain are paralysed, and in which the voluntary motions are almost suspended for want of convolutional stimulus, but where the patients usually retain the power of standing, walking, masticating and swallowing."

It must be distinctly understood that stupor is not in itself a disease but only a symptom in the course of a disease, that it may complicate any mental disorder, and occurs as a definite stage in the course of all cases of katatonia. It may present varying characters during the course of a single case, and hence to treat it as a condition apart and subdivide it up, as many authors do, is most confusing, for in by far the larger number of cases one condition passes into another; the non-resistive case of to-day may be the resistive one to-morrow, etc., etc.

It is much more commonly seen in adolescence than during adult life and varies greatly in severity and type. Thus there may be complete loss of consciousness and memory, or the patient may remain wholly conscious and remember clearly everything which occurred during his illness. In all cases of stupor there is impaired nutrition, alimentary disturbance, and defective circulation with marked loss of muscular tone leading to cyanosed and œdematous extremities. All cases of stupor must be carefully watched as they are liable to sudden impulses which may be of a destructive, homicidal or suicidal character.

Mental Enfeeblement may be primary, *i.e.*, congenital, in origin (imbecility, idiocy, primary dementia or amentia) or secondary to acute mental disease, or be due to the natural failure of the mental powers in old age. It may be a transient condition resulting from ill-health or nervous exhaustion from severe illness, shock, or physical or mental strain. It may be prominent as the result of cerebral lesions caused by accident, vascular changes, etc. It is met with in very varying degrees, from a mere blunting of the intelligence up to complete fatuity, and may imply loss of judgment, of will power and of self-control, blunting of the moral sense, impairment of the memory, loss of the powers of imagination and of attention and interest, all these being variously affected in every case, sometimes singly, sometimes in groups and in all degrees.

Self-control is perhaps the one faculty which may be said to be essential for sanity and loss of which characterises a man as insane. Even here one cannot dogmatise, however, for, as with every other mental process, so it is with this, and all shades of its enfeeblement are matters of every-day occurrence, from the merely passionate man up to the acutely excited maniac who tears up everything he can reach, shouts, laughs, grimaces and sings without any cause whatsoever. Each case must be judged on its own merits here. Thus it is absurd to expect the same self-control from a child as from an adult, from a person in health as from one pulled down by illness and suffering. Still it is a point which should invariably be looked for and estimated in all cases, for, though of great diagnostic importance as an early symptom of mental breakdown, yet more often than not it is either overlooked or misinterpreted.

Impulsiveness, another common characteristic of the insane, is directly due to the loss of self-control, and may be defined as the committing of an action consciously but without motive or forethought, even though the action is at times directly opposed by the will power of the person committing it.

Impulses may be either of reflex or central origin. Thus they may be stimulated in the former case by hallucinations of sight or hearing, while in the latter case the impulse is purely central or cortical in origin and arises apparently without cause and quite unexpectedly.

The impulses may be of varied forms, those most commonly met with being impulses to destroy anything and everything, to steal and to commit homicide or suicide. In some cases the patient feels the onset of the impulse and calls out to those around to bind him or restrain him from committing the act he is feeling impelled to do, and, if not at once restrained, it is a certainty that in a very short time, perhaps a few seconds, the act whose performance he dreaded will have been carried out.

The faculty of attention is variously affected in the insane. In some it is entirely *subjective*, every thought being occupied by the feelings of misery, depression or sensory disturbances, while not a thought, not a glance is given to what is passing around them. In other cases, as in the excited stage of folie circulaire, the attention is wholly *objective* being attracted by every movement or sound. Again, as in stupor and confüsed conditions, there is complete abolition of attention, the patient paying no heed to his own feelings and sensations any more than he does to what is passing around him. In acute toxic conditions both subjective and objective attention are impaired and the capacity for work is in abeyance. This is also the chief mental symptom in hebephrenia, where there is complete loss of these as well as incapacity to work or even to join in amusements. Similar conditions are noted in varying extent as a sequel to all the acute insanities, and are often the first indications of the onset of secondary dementia.

Change in **Sexual Desire** is often seen in many forms of insanity. Usually a primary eroticism and a subsequent temporary or permanent loss of the sexual instinct is seen in most of such cases. The former condition often leads to shameless acts of indecency.

The **Æsthetic and Religious Instincts** are often affected, becoming diminished or perverted according to the type of insanity. In old-standing cases they may form a source of delusions which become the most prominent features of the case.

Volition is variously affected in mental disorders. It may be entirely lost, as in secondary dementia where there is loss of power to originate action or new ideas in varying extent. In some cases of depression and confusion volition seems to be paralysed and such patients can never decide on their course of action and everything becomes a source of doubt and indecision. In other cases again the derangement is seen as extreme obstinacy and resistiveness to every action suggested, though if the same action originate spontaneously it is readily and voluntarily performed.

Memory both near and distant is more or less impaired in all states of confusion and loss of consciousness. In states of mental depression or exhaustion memory remains, but its use is a distinct effort to the patient and it rapidly becomes exhausted, while in certain other conditions, as in the elevated stage of folie circulaire, the memory is abnormally active for both near and distant events. A failure of memory for recent events alone is characteristic of senile and alcoholic cases. At times a condition of "false memory," or *paramnesia,* is met with, which is really more properly classifiable under the term Delusion.

Speech, though it really originates, strictly speaking, in the motor centres, is so closely connected with all mental processes that it is usually implicated in the course of insanity. In states of excitement it is profuse, loud and tumultuous, just as other motor centres through overaction cause restlessness and exaggerated muscular movements. From its mental aspect in these cases the speech is incoherent or disconnected, and the association of ideas accidental or fragmentary.

The mental condition too is often indicated by the character of the speech. Thus when delusions of grandeur and exaggerated self-importance are present the speech is pompous and boastful, as in general paralysis of the insane, and in states of depression the speech is much diminished and everything said is enunciated in scarcely audible whispers. In complete stupor speech is entirely in abeyance, while in less marked stupor, as is met with in katatonia, the implication of the speech centre is seen in verbigeration, or a repetition of numbers, words or sentences in a rhythmical manner, and in echolalia or imitation of the words and tone of anyone speaking in the hearing of the patient.

Incoherence may be due to confusion and result in a tumultuous rush of words without any marked cortical change being present, as in conditions of acute excitement, or it may be due directly to functional or structural changes in the grey matter.

Impairment of speech too may be directly due to muscular paresis as in G. P. I.

The *handwriting* often changes in character during attacks of insanity, being as a rule larger and bolder during excitement and elevation, with copious underlinings and numerous exclamation marks. Indeed at times the pen seems almost to "take charge," every available piece of paper being written on and sometimes crossed and recrossed two or three times. In states of depression it is as a rule thin, small and straggling.

Disturbances of the emotions are very common in the insane, and indeed in certain types of insanity form the chief symptoms of the malady. Thus patients suffering from general paralysis of the insane and certain other forms of insanity are often unduly irritable, violent outbursts of passion occurring with little or even no provocation. In other cases the emotions seem to be in a condition of unstable equilibrium, the patients laughing one minute and perhaps crying the next without any apparent cause, as is commonly seen in states of acute mania. As a general rule, a tendency to hysterical weeping in men is of very grave prognostic import. In melancholia, on the other hand, the emotions seem to be dulled or even in complete abeyance, failing to respond to even the strongest stimuli, a mother perhaps hearing apparently unmoved of the death of her favourite child.

Fear and constant anxiety are symptoms often met with in many types of mental derangement.

With the onset of secondary dementia the emotions fail along with the other functions of the brain and complete apathy is found as a rule in most dements whether the condition be primary or secondary.

Jealousy is a common symptom of insanity and most trying to those who have the misfortune to be its victims.

It is a frequent symptom of alcoholic insanities and in these may at times lead to homicidal attacks on the wife or her supposed paramour.

It is seen at its most extravagant heights, however, in that form of delusional insanity commonly known as "ovarian or old maid's insanity." Widows and old maids, as a rule, are the sufferers here, fixing their affections on some man, as a rule a clergyman or famous musician or actor, and dogging his footsteps and pestering him with their attentions in a most shameless manner and in spite of open rebuffs. Many a man has been seriously compromised by a woman of this type, for the ordinary laity do not understand such cases, and as the women are often cunning enough to conceal their actions, and do not otherwise exhibit any marked eccentricity, the public always shows a disposition to champion the cause of the woman, pointing the finger of scorn at the unhappy object of her attentions and hounding him out of society. To anyone having the misfortune to fall into such a predicament, my advice is to acquaint the friends of the woman at once with the annoyance caused by her conduct and to keep carefully all letters received and copies of all letters written.

Sleep is the function of the body most liable to disturbance in physical disorders, and similarly in mental disorders one may say no case occurs in which there is not some derangement of this function. This loss of the power to sleep is one of the most troublesome symptoms one has to deal with in asylums. In some cases of chronic excitement sleep is apparently absolutely abolished, and though they may be kept under observation for years, they will never be found asleep; in these cases, however, the probability is that sleep does occur, but is of so slight a character that the slightest sound rouses the patient.

In other cases there is a regular periodicity to be noted; thus the patient may sleep one night and not the next, or sleep for two nights and miss the third, and in some of these cases alterations of pulse and temperature may be noted on the day preceding or following the sleepless night.

Excessive sleep is seen at times and is specially seen in some stages of G. P. I., also during the stupor of katatonia and in some cases of epileptic insanity. Senile cases, as a rule, sleep heavily during the day and awake to abnormal activity at night.

The causes of general sleeplessness are innumerable. Very commonly it is due to a "bad brain habit" and nothing more, and in these cases a hot bath and a glass of hot milk taken just before going to bed often work marvels. In acute insanities, however, it is generally due to a toxæmia, and as the case becomes more chronic, there is superadded the acquisition of a "bad brain habit." In some cases the sleeplessness is due to the direct action of the toxine on the cortical grey matter, but in others, as shown by Dr. Bruce, the condition is due to tne production of a high arterial tension and a rapid pulse rate, which of themselves alone are capable of producing sleeplessness.

Dr. Bruce states: "The normal arterial pressure, according to Hill, is about 110 mm. Hg. with the patient in a horizontal posture. In patients who have recovered from attacks of insanity I have found the tension to vary from 100—120 mm. Hg. Another characteristic of the arterial pressure in health is that it is always lower in the evening than in ths morning. In natural sleep it was found that the arterial tension fell some 10 mm. Hg., *i.e.*, a patient who before sleep registered 110 mm. Hg., during sleep registered 100 mm. Hg. The same patient after a dose of one drachm of paraldehyde fell asleep an hour later and the arterial tension registered 80 mm. Hg. Two hours later the pressure had risen to 95 mm. Hg. and 4 hours later to 100 mm. Hg.; that is to say, during the drug sleep the arterial pressure at first fell below that of normal sleep, but gradually rose again and the drug sleep apparently passed into a condition of normal sleep.''

In addition to this it should be remembered that there is a regularly recurring rise and fall in the blood-pressure, the whole period which this cycle takes lasting about 4 weeks, and occurring not only in women, in whom it seems in some way connected with the process of menstruation, but also in men, and it is possible that this too may have some effect in producing attacks of recurrent insanity and also in the production of the various stages of folie circulaire.

Dr. Bruce further states: "In all cases of insanity suffering from metabolic poisoning and sleeplessness the arterial pressure in the evening was higher than that of the morning and during the state of sleeplessness was as high as 140—150 mm. Hg., but if sleep occurred naturally, the tension always fell below 110 mm. Hg. In a similar condition sleep induced by such a drug as paraldehyde was accompanied by a fall in pressure to at least 110 mm. Hg., but rarely lower. In patients suffering from excitement a high arterial tension was often associated with the state of sleeplessness and in these cases also the arterial pressure always fell, whether sleep occurred normally or by the use of drugs. It was found, however, that some patients suffering from excitement with sleeplessness—particularly from excited melancholia—had abnormally low arterial pressures with a rapid pulse rate. In such cases the exhibition of, say, two drachms of paraldehyde raised the pressure and further excited the patient while doses of 10—15 min. of paraldehyde, 30 grs. of sulphonal or 20 grs. of trional lowered the pulse rate and produced sleep without in any way altering the arterial pressure.'' This should be carefully noted as the pulse tension and rate are really most excellent indicators of what sedative to use and in what dose, and my small experience, about 12 years, had led me to very much this line of action though without having carried out the observations so carefully noted by Dr. Bruce.*

---

* Studies in Clinical Psychiatry by Lewis C. Bruce, M.D., F.R.C.P.E., q.v.

CHAPTER V.

PHYSICAL SYMPTOMS.

If not in all, at least in by far the majority of cases of insanity, there are well-marked physical symptoms in addition to those of mental derangement. These in most cases precede the onset of any mental disturbance, and, if rightly interpreted and treated by the medical attendant, an attack of insanity may in many cases be averted. This point has always seemed to me a most important one and it has surprised me to find it slurred over, as it is, in so many standard books on insanity. I would therefore impress on my readers as far as possible the necessity of being able to read and interpret aright these symptoms, and will endeavour to give them what help and assistance I can in this way, as concisely as possible.

Alimentary System.—As already stated, many of the cases of insanity due to bacillary toxæmia arise from bacilli normally habitant in the alimentary canal. Hence it is a natural sequence to say that in many forms of insanity the alimentary canal is found to be deranged in some way, and that if this condition be treated, an improvement of the mental symptoms is noted.

Carious teeth are common adjuncts among the inmates of asylums even at home, and, in India, from the little experience I have had, I should say much more prevalent than among the same classes outside of asylums, and in such cases the removal of the teeth and proper treatment of the septic buccal conditions often causes marked improvement in the mental symptoms.

A furred or coated tongue, indicative of dyspepsia, is nearly always seen in the acute insanities, and a dry, brown, cracked tongue is an invariable concomitant of insanity due to exhaustion or septicæmia which has passed into the typhoid state.

The appetite for food and liquids is practically always lost in the acute insanities, and is a common call for artificial feeding. In most of such cases there is a failure in the secretion of digestive juices, and I have frequently seen such patients vomit a meal of eggs, milk and meat juice practically unchanged even two hours after injection through the feeding tube. In cases of acute melancholia or mania the gastric juice, when withdrawn, has practically no action on food-stuffs even when left in contact for two hours or more. Thus the first and an important point to note is that dyspepsia with all its symptoms is a common concomitant of, and may often precede, any of the acute insanities.

Hæmopoietic System.—The *thyroid gland* has been proved through the experiments of Horsley and others to have undoubted and important relations with nervous diseases. Thus its complete removal in such an animal as the monkey causes a condition practically indistinguishable from the disease in man known as myxœdema, and conversely if a case of myxœdema be treated with thyroid extract marked improvement invariably ensues. The chief mental condition in myxœdema is of hebetude and many cases of insanity characterised by a listless inertia react most wonderfully to a course of thyroid extract. It is also at times of great use in cases of depression, excitement or elevation, due probably to deficient or altered secretion of the thyroid. Such cases, however, are very hard to distinguish, and in the majority of them the treatment is begun tentatively at first and only continued if good results follow its exhibition. At times too I have seen the depression much increased and at others an almost maniacal condition produced by this course of treatment.

Leucocytes as shown by recent bacteriological research are increased in number, above those normally present in the blood, in certain toxic conditions and to this increase the term hyperleucocytosis is applied. This increase is not proportional in each and every type of leucocyte, but especially effects the polymorphonuclear elements which in health normally amount to about 60% of the 7,000 or more leucocytes as a whole present per c.mm. In toxic conditions the leucocytosis may rise as high as 30,000 per c.mm. or even higher, and the polymorphonuclears may increase to as much as 90% of the whole.

In addition to these corpuscular changes during toxæmias there is also the formation, in the blood, of *alexines* or substances capable of neutralising the toxic bodies present, and, when in addition to toxines we have to deal with the presence of bacteria in the blood-stream, there are certain other bodies present, of which the chief one for our purpose is known as an "agglutinine." These substances have the power of clumping the organism causing the infection when mixed with it in vitro, *e.g.*, Widal's reaction for typhoid fever.

Dr. Bruce has examined the blood of many cases of acute insanity for bacteria, but in only two was he successful in obtaining an organism. One, a case of acute mania in a typhoid state, gave a pure growth of a small streptococcus, and the other, a case of katatonia, yielded a somewhat larger streptococcus. He tested the serum reaction of 23 cases of mania with both these organisms in dilutions of 1—30 and in 19 cases obtained definite agglutination of the organism obtained from the case of acute mania. The serum of 6 cases of excited melancholia similarly tested gave agglutination of the same organism in 3 cases. Twelve cases of katatonia when tested with the larger organism gave a definite reaction in 6 cases.

Another point noted by Dr. Bruce, and one well worth remembering, is that for the production of agglutinines it is not essential that the organism should be present in the blood-stream, the mere digestion of the organisms in the stomach sufficing to produce this effect in a healthy animal. Hence it is probable that in many cases the source of trouble may be in the naso-pharynx or indeed any part of the alimentary canal, even the large intestine, for absorption takes place largely from it, and Ford Robertson has pointed out that atrophic changes in the mucous and sub-mucous coats of the large intestine are common in all forms of acute insanity which present symptoms of toxæmia and also in cases of general paralysis.

Red bone marrow has been examined by Dr. Bruce from cases which showed hyperleucocytosis in life, and in every case he found the marrow was leucoblastic and the cells undergoing active mytotic division.

Circulatory System.—The *heart* in the insane shows, on the whole, a larger percentage of valvular lesions than in the sane, and the onset of valvular incompetence, especially in old people, is frequently followed by mental symptoms.

The main circulatory accompaniment of insanity, however, is altered *arterial tension*, which may be increased or diminished, the former being more usually a concomitant of states of depression and the latter of states of excitement or elevation. In health the arterial tension is as a rule about 115 mm. Hg., but in nervous derangements it may rise to 160—170 mm., according to Bruce, or fall well below 100 mm. Hg.

Pulse changes are best seen in acute melancholia when a pulse rate of 120 per minute may be associated with a temperature of 99°F. or even less. In acute mania a fast weak pulse with sub-normal temperature may be one of the earliest symptoms. In cases of stupor the tension and pulse rate fall enormously, the latter falling as low as 50 beats per minute or even less and, with this, failure in peripheral circulation is shown by cold feet and œdematous extremities.

Respiratory System.—As phthisis has been noted as a predisposing cause of insanity, so conversely the diminished vitality so common among the insane renders them more than ordinarily liable to phthisis.

In general paralysis Ford Robertson, McRae and Jeffrey have recently discovered a bacillus in the lungs which when eaten by the rat produces a slowly progressive paralysis terminating in death. Bruce repeated this experiment on a goat, with death as a result from paralytic symptoms, more than one year after infection, the infection occurring through the alimentary tract, the goat having licked the site of injection.

Integument.—Changes in the hair, the skin and the nails are practically invariable concomitants of all types of insanity. Patients in the acute phases of the disease do not as a rule complain of subjective symptoms, but irritations of the skin and the scalp must be undoubtedly common, judging by the numbers who pull out their hair, scratch and wash their heads on every available opportunity. The cause is difficult to explain, but, if we theorise, the only three tenable explanations seem to be trophic changes due to implication of peripheral nerves or their centres, or a hyperexcitability of sensory nerves due to peripheral or central changes, or lastly, the condition may be due to altered secretion causing irritation.

In support of the first of these theories we have the appearance of pigmentary deposits, and the occurrence of phagedenic ulcers, both of which are common experiences in asylum practice. In support of the second it is not so easy to bring forward proof though at times one meets with cases where, though the integument is absolutely normal in appearance, the patient constantly complains of insects running over or beneath the skin, or of having needles stuck into her, and there can be but little doubt, I think, that these delusions arise from disordered sensory nerves. The third of these theories can be readily proved by the dry hard skin seen in melancholics owing to deficient excretion of the waste products in the body, or the drenching perspirations seen at times in katatonia, or as a crisis in acute mania. A crop of boils sometimes occurs during the invasion period of an attack of acute mania, and as a rule such a condition can be looked on as indicative of a favourable prognosis.

In by far the greater number of cases of insanity, if not in all, the hair and nails become dry and brittle, and in some cases of mania the hair more or less stands on end giving a finishing touch to the appearance characteristic of such conditions.

Urinary System.—The frequency of the act of micturition depends on two separate causes, firstly, on the amount of urine excreted; and secondly, on the centre in the brain concerned in the reflex act of micturition being in a fit state to receive sensory impressions from the bladder and transpose them into the origination of the act. The first condition is well exemplified in cases of acute melancholia where there is a suppression of urinary excretion and but little urine is voided as a result, usually from 8-9 oz. in 24 hours, though at times less. In cases where consciousness is impaired the act of micturition may be delayed solely through the inability of the cortical centres to respond to the stimuli received from a full bladder, and in such cases a careful watch should be kept for the necessity of catheterisation as the excretion of urine is in no way diminished.

Albuminuria is frequently met with, especially in cases of mania and melancholia, and as a rule is due to irritation as numerous leucocytes can be found microscopically in the urine. Very occasionally it is due to vasomotor disturbances.

Glycosuria, which is occasionally seen after epileptic fits and in delusional conditions, is invariably vasomotor in origin.

The Excretion of Chlorides is diminished in certain cases of toxæmic origin.

Reproductive System.—*Menstruation* among insane women, especially adolescents in Europe, is usually most irregular, by far the majority of them suffering from amenorrhœa. When menstruation, however, does occur it is as a rule accompanied by relapses and exacerbations in the mental symptoms, and no case can be said to have completely recovered till this function has become regular and normal in its occurrence. In India, however, so far as my experience goes, menstruation among the female inmates of asylums seems to correspond fairly closely with what one meets with in the same classes among the sane population, both as regards the number of the periods and the quantity of flow at each period (*vide* Chap. 20).

Masturbation is still regarded by many as one of the concomitant exciting causes of insanity. This view is now becoming a thing of the past, and rightly too, for, though it may tend to weaken the patient and exaggerate the mental symptoms, there can be but little doubt that in most cases masturbation is merely an early symptom and due to impairment of the higher controlling centres of the brain allowing lower centres to come more into evidence.

The Testicles and Ovaries undoubtedly play an important part in the developement and nutrition of the body and mind. Their removal in either sex before the completion of developement causes complete arrest of the formation of both the bodily and mental sexual characteristics, and it is just possible, as suggested by Dr. Bruce, that deficient or altered secretory activity may co-exist with an apparently, but not really, healthy state of these organs and be the cause of the symptoms of arrested developement seen so commonly in cases of insanity occurring during puberty and adolescence. Certain forms of insanity, such as "ovarian insanity" and "old maid's insanity," have been said to arise from derangement of the uterus and ovaries, but no proof has ever been adduced to show that there is even a connection between the conditions.

Vasomotor and Nutritional Disturbances are common in all forms of insanity. *Inequality of the axillary temperatures* occurs at times in cases of general paralysis, katatonia and melancholia. In the first it generally occurs after congestive seizures more or less unilateral in character, but in the two last no such explanation is possible and one has just to accept it as an undoubted fact.

Extremely low temperatures, seen in the course of mania, excited melancholia and katatonia, are probably due to vasomotor disturbances, while the flushing of the cheeks characteristic of the onset of mania, and pallor and lividity, seen in cases of stupor, acute melancholia and at times dementia, are due to similar causes.

Excessive Perspiration may be either reflex in origin, as in the course of acute insanity, when it probably is due to fear caused by terrifying hallucinations or delusions, or it may be a direct effort of nature to eliminate poisons from the system, as so often occurs in cases of katatonia or at the crisis of mania and melancholia. At times unilateral perspiration occurs in katatonia especially after taking food, but the cause of this is unknown.

Lachrymal Secretion is often suppressed, and one of the most extraordinary sights in an asylum is to see a patient wandering hither and thither, wringing his hands, sobbing and crying in an agony of grief, without there being a trace even of a tear visible. In such cases often the first sign of improvement is a flood of tears and the restoration of the lachrymal secretion.

Salivation may be modified and, as a rule, when affected it is in excess, though how much is really in excess and how much only apparent and due to diminished reflexes causing its collection in, and flow from the mouth is rather hard to decide.

The Nervous System from which one would expect to obtain most information in this class of cases, is as a rule the most difficult to examine owing to the patients being unable to afford us any assistance. In those forms of mental disease where consciousness is impaired it is impossible to test *sensation* owing to the inability of the patient to realise pain, *i.e.*, the loss of subject-consciousness.

In certain forms of delusional insanity, such as those due to alcoholic excess, sensations of tingling and formication often give rise to delusions of a persecutory character, such as "electrical agencies," "hypnotism," or vermin in the bed or garments. In the few cases that can be tested, sensation is variously affected. It may be deficient or hyperacute, sense of heat may be lost, etc., etc., and these symptoms are in no way connected with any type of the disease and are therefore no aid to diagnosis.

In folie circulaire the sense of sight at times varies enormously in the different stages, thus you may have normal vision in the stage of elevation, but gradually as depression sets in stronger and stronger glasses are required, as pointed out by Clouston. Similarly the other special senses may be affected, giving rise to various delusions and hallucinations, such as unseen people abusing the patient, poisoned food, the presence of noxious vapours in the air, etc., etc.

The pupils are variously affected in insanity. Inequality of the pupils is common in various forms of insanity, especially in cases of long standing. In conditions of excitement, exhaustion or fear the pupils are widely dilated and react sluggishly both to light and accommodation. In general paralysis, in senile cases where there are degenerative changes in the cortex, and in excited cases in a state of anger there are nearly always pinpoint pupils, though not invariably, as at times the pupil in general paralysis may be widely dilated.

Where consciousness is impaired control of the reflex acts of *defœcation and micturition* is lost and uncleanliness results. This is not always the cause of uncleanliness, however, as often in cases of dementia it is due to a loss of the ordinary instincts of cleanliness and the patient can be re-educated to more cleanly habits.

Swallowing is at times impaired, where there is loss of sensibility, or advanced muscular paresis as in general paralysis. Its impairment in katatonia, where the saliva often dribbles from the mouth, is due to an extension of the state of "passive resistance" to this function as the reflex is not in any way abolished and it is customary to feed such cases by hand and not by the tube.

The Superficial reflexes are increased in all cases where there is a loss of consciousness as in acute mania. They are decreased in cases where the reflex arc is severed as in alcoholic cases, or in cases of stupor where there is increased cerebral inhibition. *Deep reflexes* do not necessarily follow this rule, as there may be no increase in the kneejerk in cases characterised by loss of consciousness. The tendon reflexes are increased as a rule in the first stage of general paralysis, in certain cases of stupor, especially katatonic stupor, and in old standing epileptics; like the superficial reflexes they are diminished in cases where the reflex arc is interfered with.

Paresis of the voluntary muscles is seldom met with except in advanced general paralysis, organic and secondary dementia, traumatic insanity and certain variations of senile insanity. *Inco-ordination* is, however, present in all acute insanities, from mere failure of finely associated movements to the wild purposeless movements of acute excitement. Mere sluggishness of movement, characteristic of hebephrenia and certain cases of melancholia, is due to deficient volition and no implication of the cortical motor areas can be demonstrated as a rule.

All mentalisation arises primarily from three prime factors, the *reception of motion*, the *modification of motion* and *the emission of motion*, corresponding to Sensation, Thought and Will respectively. Similarly all motor phenomena in the body may be said to arise from impulses from the central nervous system, *i.e.*, are mental in origin. Thus it can be readily seen how complex their relation is.

During *sleep*, where consciousness is lost, there is a relegation of nervous activity to the spinal centres, a negative activity of the higher centres, accompanied by a relatively, but not absolutely, increased activity of the lower centres, and muscular tonus is lost. On awakening from sleep, with the return of consciousness, the brain regaining control over the lower reflex centres sends down a steady flow of energy and tonus returns. Similar conditions prevail in varying degree when one feels out of form or conversely "as fit as a fiddle," and in each of these conditions the mental state is depicted in every movement and attitude of the body.

Attention, as with other forms of mentalisation, is closely associated with motion. Thus it originates in motion, requiring some form of motion, either sound waves or light rays, to stimulate it. It also is the cause of the emission of motion as can be easily seen by watching a person engrossed, say, in a lecture, his muscular tonus is increased, especially that of the muscles of expression, the orbicularis muscles being tense and the eyes directed towards the object exciting the attention and involuntarily tracing its outlines and originating thus sensations tending to fix the impression on the cortex.

Similarly *Memory*, *Will* and *Speech* can all be shown to be closely connected with motor phenomena. From this it can be readily understood why in health the mental condition is reflected in the expression, the attitude, the actions of the subject. In mental disease this condition still holds good and is even at times enormously exaggerated, *e.g.*, in melancholiacs where the motor manifestations are often palpably out of all proportion to the state of mental depression felt by the patient.

CHAPTER VI.

GENERAL PATHOLOGY.

THE recent work of Lewis C. Bruce, M.D., F.R.C.P.E., has largely revolutionised the views previously held in this branch of psychiatry, and has given an impetus to research in a new direction which, I think, at no distant date will bring forth invaluable knowledge as to the cause of the majority of the forms of insanity. As a result specific treatment on serum-therapeutical lines will probably arise for cases where at present the best that can be done is to treat them on sound hygienic principles, and endeavour to improve the condition by suitable feeding and employment, as well for the body as the mind.

Up till late years alienists as a rule were content with finding gross lesions, such as thickening of the membranes, congestions of localised areas of brain tissue, atheromatous arteries or various degenerations of cortical nerve cells, and bringing forth these as the causes of the various forms of insanity. It never seemed to strike them that such pathological changes could not originate *de novo*, that there must be some cause for such changes, and that any cause capable of producing such marked changes on comparatively gross tissues, would in all probability be capable of exerting a still greater effect on the highly specialised structures in the cortex, which, though not perhaps capable of demonstration microscopically, would still account largely for many of the conditions to be found in any of our asylums.

That these gross lesions exist and have an effect on the mental symptoms is undoubtedly true. To say that they have any effect in producing any one class of symptoms, *i.e.*, that any one, or indeed any group, of such pathological lesions is universally characteristic of any one type of insanity, is a fallacy which is daily becoming more apparent. Normal brains show such widely different reactions to exactly the same stimuli, that it is only to be expected, and is indeed the case, that a still greater difference lies between the response of unstable brains to exactly similar conditions.

GROSS PATHOLOGICAL CHANGES.

The Cranial Bones may be uniformly increased in density, or this increase may occur in irregular patches, or the converse conditions may be found and they may be reduced to an extraordinary degree of tenuity.

At times from degenerative causes they may be unduly friable, and the cancellated tissue may vary in appearance according to whether anæmic or congestive conditions have been present. Increased density with adhesions of the dura mater is commonly seen in cases of chronic insanity and epilepsy.

The Dura Mater may be the seat of various lesions. Thickening with adhesion to the skull-cap is of common occurrence. Inflammations, with exudates and hæmorrhages, may occur and form cysts and discoloured patches, and at times adhesions between dura and pia mater denote inflammations of the serous surfaces of these membranes. Except as they affect the venous or lymphatic circulation through the pia however, and thus react upon the nutrition of the brain substance, none of these lesions are of much significance.

Lesions of the Pia Mater are, however, of much greater import, as into its meshes flows by far the larger portion of the blood and lymph from the brain. The most serious, and a fairly frequent, pathological condition is that known as *gelatinous thickening*, which is due to a congestion of the lymph flow, and causes atrophy of the cerebral tissue. (A certain amount of pial cloudiness is practically physiological in all persons over middle age, and must not be mistaken for a pathological condition). In such cases the membrane is thickened and of a gelatinous consistence, the thickening being most marked over the vertex and in the neighbourhood of the Pacchionian bodies. On close examination along the course of dilated arteries and veins the dilated lymph channels can be seen as a fine bluish white line, which is absolutely characteristic of this condition, which it must be remembered is of a purely degenerative type. As the condition progresses the lymph channels become more and more occluded until finally the whole brain becomes bathed with the dammed up waste products, many of which are undoubtedly poisonous, and in this way atrophy and degeneration of neuroglia and nerve cells are produced as the final result.

Hæmorrhages into the pia are of fairly common occurrence and may form hæmorrhagic cysts. They occur as a rule over the vertex, and are frequently associated with mental symptoms.

Inflammatory conditions are generally associated with dense adhesions between the brain substance and meninges, so that it is often impossible to separate them. This "meningo-cerebritis" resembles in appearance more an advanced degree of gelatinous thickening than an inflammatory process, and in many cases it is only by the presence of adhesions to the cerebrum that one can distinguish between them by the naked eye. Rupture of a pial artery followed by extensive hæmorrhage is of very rare occurrence, and, when it does occur, is as a rule rapidly fatal.

Gross Lesions of the Brain Substance are common in many, but characteristic of no special form of mental disease. In chronic insanities atrophy of the entire cortex, with serous exudation and gelatinous thickening of the pia mater, is practically always present.

Thrombosis and embolism are common causes of localised atrophies, which may also result from arterio-sclerosis or the occlusion of arteries as a sequel of syphilitic disease.

Hyperæmic conditions are evidenced *post-mortem* by vascular dilatations, and varicose-like conditions of arteries and veins may be seen at times. Anæmic conditions, which are as a rule more commonly met with, may result from thickening of arterial sheaths.

Inflammation of the brain substance is very rare indeed as a local condition, and when present is generally due to thrombus, or cancerous or tubercular growths. The site of the lesion is generally pinker than the surrounding healthy brain substance, though occasionally the converse is seen and the affected area is much paler.

Atrophy of the Hemispheres is found *post-mortem* after all forms of chronic insanity, after the senile psychoses and chronic alcoholism. It consists of atrophy affecting both the gray and the white matter, and though as a rule diffuse, may at times be found localised in one or more lobes. It usually affects the cortex, medullary matter and basal ganglia about equally, the result being that the gray matter is perceptibly reduced in thickness and the ventricles are more or less dilated, owing to shrinkage of the white medulla without as a rule any compensatory granulation of the ependyma or dilatation of the choroid plexuses. The convolutions are found to be thin and pointed as a rule in such cases though at times, if there be much serous exudation, they may be found to be flattened. *Microscopically* degeneration of the neuroglia is found to be present, the star-rayed elements being relatively increased owing to the disappearance of the other elements, and the nerve fibres present a varicose appearance. The nerve cells likewise show signs of degeneration and are often pigmented.

Localised atrophy is seen in some cases of paretic dementia, or one hemisphere may be affected more than the other in such cases. When it occurs it is most frequent in the frontal lobes, the motor areas and occipital region coming next in frequency. At times patches of marked atrophy may be seen surrounded by apparently healthy gyri, and such cases are as a rule due to obstruction of an artery from some cause, or more rarely to a localised inflammation.

The Degenerations of the Nerve Cells have been, and are even up to the present time, a fruitful source of discussion among pathologists and others, owing to the great difficulty there is in distinguishing lesions the result of disease, from lesions occurring in the preparation of the specimen. This difficulty, however, is being gradually removed, and we are by degrees becoming more and more able to distinguish a true from an artificial lesion.

During the last 15 years or so three distinct methods have been employed in this research :—

1. *Nissl's alcohol-methylene-blue method ;* 2. *The chrome-silver method and its modifications ;* 3. *Ordinary hardening with alcohol, etc., and staining by ordinary aniline dyes, hæmatoxylene, carmine, etc.* It is beyond the scope, however, of this book to go into these processes minutely, and a mere summary of the degenerations most commonly met with will be given here. Those requiring further information on this subject will do well in consulting the text-books either of Bevan Lewis or Berkley.

Fatty Degeneration is the most common pathological condition of the nerve cell found *post-mortem,* and must be distinguished from the yellowish granules found normally in the large cells of the cortex after middle age, and whose true origin and nature are not as yet definitely known. In true fatty degeneration the pigment granules undergo an immense increase in numbers, and, pushing the nucleus before them, ultimately occupy by far the larger part of the cell. At this stage the outline of the cell is ill-defined and the cell itself has enlarged and undergone alteration in its shape. Later the nucleus, which remains practically unchanged in the first stage, rejects the basic stains but takes up acid stains with avidity, later still its vesicular outline is lost, it becomes angular, stains deeply and shows in its centre a bright refractile spot. Should degeneration advance still further, the nucleus shrinks, the pigment granules become a brownish colour, the protoplasm is absorbed and finally the pigment granules are found lying loose in the intercellular space. This condition is common in congestive conditions, or where there is obstruction of the circulation in any way.

Simple Atrophy of the Cell is commonly seen in anæmic conditions, such as ensue after thrombus or embolism. The cell shrinks, its processes become angular, and the nucleus gradually becoming roughened, eccentric and indistinct, finally wholly disappears, and the cell undergoes absorption.

Coarse Granular Degeneration is at times seen after inflammatory processes. The cell swells up and loses its definition, while coarse granular masses, staining readily with logwood or carmine, gather round the nucleus which becomes eccentric and at times even extruded from the body of the cell.

Vacuolation of the Protoplasm may be either due to *post-mortem* changes or the result of disease, but is generally due to the former causes and of but little importance. It is sometimes, but not invariably, found in epilepsy, and usually also occurs after intense stimulation by an eléctric current.

Colloid Degeneration is generally found in localised inflammations or in the neighbourhood of old-standing hæmorrhages. The cell is tumefied and the colloid masses stain deeply with carmine or logwood.

Depigmentation and Hyaline Degeneration are closely allied to each other and intimately associated with sclerotic changes in the cell substance. The granular appearance of the cell substance disappears, dyes are less and less readily taken up, the protoplasm becomes homogeneous, the cell barely distinguishable from the surrounding matrix, and finally complete atrophy ensues.

Finely Granular Degeneration of the Cell is fairly common and usually accompanies toxæmic conditions. The cells become tumefied, the protoplasm granular and stains are but feebly taken up even by the nucleus, which itself becomes shrunken, distorted and eccentric. The condition seems to be akin to a fatty degeneration, as in the perivascular spaces, in addition to broken down leucocytes, there is a large amount of granular débris which blackens more or less readily with osmic acid.

Calcareous Degenerations are at times seen as the result of irritations. Cells thus affected have a bright almost iridescent appearance, owing to altered refraction, and their processes appear broken and irregular. If a drop of acid be added to the preparation, bubbles of CO_2 are evolved and characteristic crystals of the corresponding lime salts are deposited on the specimen.

Degeneration of the Nerve Fibres is mainly seen as the result of acute inflammations or irritative processes. It begins as a rule with swelling of the axis-cylinder and a varicose condition of the medullary sheath, ill-defined retrograde conditions then occur, ultimately resulting in the disappearance of the fibre.

Lesions of the Neuroglia are frequently seen in all forms of mental disease. In irritative conditions an atrophy of the cellular elements is very commonly met with, the cell bodies and processes becoming granular and tumefied, and finally breaking down and filling the perivascular spaces with a finely granular débris. The cells of the neuroglia are more resistant to toxic processes than the nerve cells, except for the long rayed spider cells which seem possessed of wonderful vitality and capable of existing under most adverse conditions.

Lesions of the Cerebral Arteries and Veins show no pathological differences to similar lesions found elsewhere in the body and for descriptions of them the reader is referred to pathological text-books, where the subject is more fully dealt with in detail than can be done in a book of this type.

CLINICAL PATHOLOGY.

Some of the most common pathological conditions have been described above and in recent years many more conditions of similar characters have been investigated, but, beyond showing that such conditions can be present, and apparently be connected with various types of insanity, we are no nearer ascertaining the cause of these pathological conditions, the true causes of the insanities, than when these histological conditions were unknown. The line of research started by Dr. Bruce, a clinical study of mental diseases, supplemented by clinical pathology and laboratory observations, is undoubtedly one full of promise and has already brought forth great results in his hands. It is from his work that most of the matter for this section has been taken, for the reason that up to date I have only been in charge of an asylum for little over a year. My work has been either under the direction of others, principally Dr. Reid of the Aberdeen Asylum, to whose kindness and instruction I owe most of my knowledge of this subject, or as specialist to the Military Department of the Government of India, where, though one necessarily keeps "au fait" with everything, one has but little material to work with, and in matters of this sort to bring forward statistics based on 20 or 30, or even 200 or 300 cases is fully as absurd as to try to vindicate a certain method of treatment on the results obtained from an epidemic of similar numbers.

1. **Temperature.**—Various types of temperature are seen in the hospital wards of modern asylums, conforming to those of similar physical diseases seen in ordinary infirmaries. There are, however, two main features in the temperatures of insane patients which are worthy of note ; firstly, that the febrile reaction is very rarely in proportion to the severity of the disease, and secondly that often with a high polymorphonuclear leucocytosis there may be no febrile temperature, *i.e.*, with every clinical evidence of a virulent toxæmia, there is no corresponding febrile reaction. Judging from my own experience both the above noted features are present, and fully as frequently seen in Indian as in Scotch Asylums.

2. **Bacteria of the Mouth and Stomach.**—Associated with all toxæmic insanities there is an accumulation, on the lips, teeth and tongue, of sordes which swarm with bacteria mainly of the streptococcus group. These streptococci are found to be extremely virulent when injected intravenously into rabbits, doses of even 0·1 c.c. having proved fatal in 3—4 hours, though the streptococci grown from the saliva of a healthy man are not markedly virulent when injected into the lower animals.

Similar results have been obtained by Bruce in cases associated with excess of bacteria in the gastric contents. Here too streptococci are preponderant and even more toxic apparently than those from the buccal sordes.

3. **Coagulation of the Blood.**—Many facts have been recently brought to light from systematic and long continued examinations of this phenomenon. Thus in katatonia and acute mania the coagulation time is immensely delayed, in some cases of katatonic stupor 20—30 minutes being required to complete coagulation.

4. **Hæmolysis** has also yielded some most interesting results under Bruce's investigations; thus he cites a case where blood serum from a case of acute mania with confusion hæmolysed the washed red blood corpuscles of a case of general paralysis when mixed in vitro in the proportion of 1 part of red blood corpuscles to 3 parts serum. The same serum mixed in the same proportion with control red blood corpuscles did not alter them in the least in six hours, while control serum mixed in the same way with the red corpuscles of the general paralytic also had no action.

5. **Leucocytosis**.—With our modern advances in knowledge, observations on leucocytosis in mental diseases have a distinctly practical bearing, as it is now known that certain diseased conditions are almost invariably associated with alterations in the number of leucocytes per c.mm. of blood and in the percentages present of the various forms of these cells. Dr. Bruce in his percentage counts, by Cole's method of counting by "fields," recognises the following forms of leucocytes :—

1. *Polymorphonuclear leucocytes*, multinucleated cells with neutrophile granules (60—70% present in normal blood).

2. *Small lymphocyte* averaging about the size of a red blood corpuscle, with a large round deeply stained nucleus surrounded by an indistinct ring of more or less granular protoplasm (20—30% normally present).

3. *Large lymphocyte* is larger than 2, and the protoplasmic ring is much more apparent (4·5—8).

4. *Hyaline or Mononuclear Leucocytes*, large cells with faintly staining protoplasm, no granules and a round or lobed nucleus which is frequently eccentric in position (3—13%).

5. *Eosinophile Leucocytes*, multinucleated cells with large eosinophile granules (1—4%).

6. *Mast Cells*, whose protoplasm contains large violet granules with a single lobed or doubled nucleus (·5—1·5%).

Total number per c.mm. in healthy men 5,000—9,000, in healthy women 6,000—13,000.

Bruce also divides his results into :—

1. *Leucocytic counts in non-toxic insanities.*

2. *Leucocytic counts in insanities due to metabolic toxæmias.*

3. *Leucocytic counts in insanities due to bacterial toxæmias.*

4. *Leucocytic counts in Epilepsy, General Paralysis and Dipsomania.*

5. *Leucocytic counts in insanities due to Alcoholic or Drug Toxæmias.*

6. *Leucocytic counts in States of Mental Enfeeblement.*

1. *Leucocytic counts in non-toxic insanities* do not call for comment. Dr. Bruce found the leucocytosis very rarely above 10,000 per c.mm. of blood; in men the polymorph percentage was generally well below 70 and in women below 60, while the large and small lymphocytes were proportionately increased. If in such cases hyperleucocytosis should occur, then the case is no longer of a pure non-toxic type, but some toxæmic condition has become superadded.

2. *In uncomplicated cases of metabolic toxæmias* hyperleucocytosis was never found. The lymphocytes are always increased in number, the polymorph percentage is as a rule low, and there is never an eosinophilia at any period. This leucocytosis seems to be unaffected by recovery or relapse. At times, however, one does see cases with a transient hyperleucocytosis and a corresponding rise in the polymorph percentage, and also a high polymorph percentage has been seen without any corresponding hyperleucocytosis. In these last two types, however, it is probable that some more

or less transitory toxæmia is the cause of the high counts, though they differ from bacterial toxæmias in that, on recovery, the hyperleucocytosis and high polymorph percentage disappears and recovery is not marked by an eosinophilia as is commonly seen in all bacterial conditions.

3. Where insanity is due to *bacterial toxæmia* there is in all cases a marked hyperleucocytosis at some period of the disease. In *excited melancholia and acute mania* it is invariably present at the onset of the disease, and is accompanied by a high polymorph percentage while eosinophiles are rarely seen. As the acute symptoms subside, there is a fall, more or less rapid, both in the leucocytosis and the percentage of the polymorphs. This fall in its turn is succeeded by a hyperleucocytosis, where however the polymorph percentage rarely rises above normal. Where recovery is rapid, this second hyperleucocytosis is as a rule rapid and accompanied by a rise in eosinophile leucocytes. In more chronic cases this hyperleucocytosis is less marked and as a rule there is an eosinophilia, these corpuscles at times amounting to 20% of the whole. A bad prognosis is indicated by a fall instead of a rise in the leucocytosis after the acute stage is over, and if the polymorphs fall below 50%, it is very bad indeed. In excited melancholia the leucocytosis is more irregular than in acute mania, and there is less tendency to a decrease in the polymorphs, *i.e.*, the toxæmia in excited melancholia has less tendency to produce secondary dementia than the toxæmia of acute mania. In recurrent attacks of either of these diseases, the leucocytosis tends to fall

just before the onset of acute symptoms and the polymorph percentage falls with it, the reaction becoming less with each recurring attack. The polymorph percentage may fall far below the average and coincidently the case may cease to be recurrent and pass into a continuous state of subacute excitement, with slight exacerbations corresponding to slight variations of the chronically persistent toxæmia.

In *folie circulaire* one sees quite a different leucocytosis. If the disease commences with a stage of elevation and is a first attack, the leucocytosis is irregular, not necessarily high, and the polymorph percentage is always well above the normal. As the elevation subsides, the leucocytosis invariably falls with it. In the depression subsequent to this elevation there is recurrent hyperleucocytosis with a relatively low polymorph percentage and frequently an eosinophilia which may last for some weeks. There is, however, no persistent hyperleucocytosis when the patient recovers. If the attack commences with depression, the hyperleucocytosis is often well marked, but the polymorph percentage rarely rises above normal. When elevation supervenes on the depression, there is first a fall in the leucocytosis and then a rise, culminating in the stage of elevation and then again falling to normal. From the above, therefore, it is evident that the toxæmia of *folie circulaire* is not persistent but fluctuating in character.

Dr. Bruce divides the leucocytosis of *katatonia* into four stages, *viz.* :—

(*a*). The leucocytosis which occurs during the acute stage of onset.

(*b*). The leucocytosis which occurs during the period of stupor.

(*c*). The leucocytosis which occurs when the patient is recovering.

(*d*). The leucocytosis of katatonic mania.

(*a*). *During the acute onset*, which rarely lasts more than three weeks, there is a marked hyperleucocytosis with an increased percentage of polymorphs as a rule, though the polymorph percentage may be unchanged. In typical cases this period terminates in a still more marked hyperleucocytosis with a greatly increased polymorph percentage. Immediately after this the patient passes into (*b*). *The stage of stupor* when the leucocytosis falls and there is a corresponding fall in the polymorph percentage, though in cases which eventually recover this percentage remains well above 65 in both sexes. A low polymorph percentage at this stage indicates a bad prognosis. Later on in the stage of stupor there occurs in most cases a slight eosinophilia, up to about 15%, and this is a hopeful sign of improvement. (*c*). If *recovery* takes place, the leucocytosis may rise and the polymorph percentage always rises above the normal average. The eosinophilia always disappears on recovery, but a slight hyperleucocytosis without any increase in the polymorph percentage is often seen in patients discharged as cured. In cases which go on to dementia a low leucocytosis and a low polymorph percentage are always present. (*d*). In cases where the *stage of stupor passes into one of mania, or maniacal* symptoms occur after a lucid interval, the leucocytosis is irregular and not marked by any increase of polymorphs or eosinophiles.

In *Hebephrenia* there is generally a slight hyper-leucocytosis with every now and then a marked rise, reaching even as high as 30,000 per c.mm. The poly-morph percentage is not necessarily high, an increase in the hyaline and large lymphocyte cells, up to 20 or 30% even, being more commonly seen. In the very rare event of a recovery taking place the leucocytosis always falls below 10,000 per c.mm.

4. In cases of *General Paralysis* the leucocytosis is of no fixed type, depending mainly on the type of mental symptoms complicating the nervous disorder. If the patient be maniacal, there is a corresponding leuco-cytosis, but if there be depression, the leucocytosis con-forms more to that of one becoming progressively weak-minded and paralysed.

If we generalise, *the first stage of G. P. I.* may be said to show an irregular hyperleucocytosis with irregular increase in the polymorph percentages and transient eosinophilias. In the *second stage*, the leucocytosis may still be irregular, but where recurrent febrile attacks are present, the leucocytosis tends to follow the tem-perature curve, and transient eosinophilias occur about the time the fever declines. In the *third stage*, the leucocytosis is markedly irregular, the polymorph per-centage is as a rule decreased, while the lymphocytes increase in numbers and may even outnumber the polymorphs. If there is a marked remission, as occasionally occurs, then the leucocytosis invariably falls below 10,000 per c.mm. of blood, and the polymorph percentage is generally very low (40—50%).

In *epileptic insanes* there is invariably a hyperleucocytosis more marked in acute than in chronic cases. In the only case of *dipsomania* examined by Dr. Bruce there was hyperleucocytosis which disappeared on recovery.

5. In *insanities due to alcohol and drug toxæmias* there was no hyperleucocytosis found.

6. In *idiots and imbeciles*, except in cases where there are symptoms of toxic insanity, such as katatonia or mania, etc., no hyperleucocytosis is found, though in *secondary dementias* irregular hyperleucocytoses are frequently seen and are as a rule associated with a low polymorph percentage.

In all insanities due to bacterial toxæmias there are certain common features in the leucocytes, noted by Dr. Bruce as follows :—

1. "During acute attacks when the leucocytosis is high and the polymorph percentage is above 70, the polymorphs are large, very granular and deeply stained and the nuclei subdivided into 5 or 6 lobes.

2. "As the acute stage passes off, the polymorphs become much less granular and their nuclei show less subdivision. Frequently an eosinophilia occurs and coincidently the granules of the polymorph cells appear to have a special affinity for the eosine dye.

3. "In patients who recover there is evidence that the leucocyte-producing cells are active, and especially the tissues which produce the polymorphonuclear cells. Such patients react vigorously to subcutaneous injections of irritants such as terebene.

4. "In patients who do not recover there is evidence that the power of polymorph production is impaired or exhausted. Such cases do not react to the subcutaneous injection of terebene or any other irritant. There is no exception to the rule that chronic cases of insanity of this class have a deficient polymorph percentage."

Agglutinines.—As already stated in Chapter V (Hæmopoietic System), agglutinines have been found by Dr. Bruce, in cases of katatonia and mania, which appear to be specific for certain varieties of streptococci isolated respectively from the blood of a case of katatonia and a case of acute mania. Adult rabbits injected with cultures of either variety of streptococcus showed more or less febrile reaction and hebetude, while rabbits of 2 or 3 days of age showed retarded developement and sooner or later developed paralysis of the hind legs, bladder and rectum. Specific agglutinines were invariably present in the blood, but in no case has either variety of streptococcus been recovered from an infected animal. Dr. Bruce prepared a vaccine from these streptococci and injected it into certain cases, with the result that in the majority of the cases specific agglutinines were found in the blood, but in no case was there any apparent benefit obtained and the treatment was discontinued.

CHAPTER VII.

CLINICAL EXAMINATION OF PATIENT.

THIS is a matter requiring infinite tact and care as an unfortunate manner, want of tact, or lack of observation may stultify the results of an examination and render you unable to certify a case when with a little care the reverse might have been the case. It is in the endeavour to give my readers a clear course of action and render this duty, difficult at all times, as easy for them as I can that I lay down the following rules for their guidance.

1. Make sure of your patient's *caste and station in life*, and learn of all you can about his caste prejudices and customs, his religious beliefs, superstitions, etc.

2. Ascertain all you can about your patient as regards heredity, temperament, habits and his behaviour generally. Go into his medical history carefully, find out how he has changed from formerly, what his delusions are, whether he is morbidly suspicious, or suicidal or homicidal. In fact, get a clear concise history of the case, noting especially the first symptoms of the case and its general course.

3. In interviews with your patient be fearless, frank, honest and a good sympathetic listener, behaving outwardly as if your patient were sane and you were treating him for some physical ailment. Do not be afraid to lead up to his weak points and delusions after you have gained his confidence. Unless you wish to test

his self-control, never contradict or irritate him and if possible avoid any sign of deceiving him. Having made sure he is ill, try and convince him of the fact too. Above all things take plenty of time and never seem in a hurry; you will only frustrate your object by doing so and far from doing yourself good may do yourself incalculable harm.

4. Note carefully his speech, manners and behaviour, how he enters the room, his bearing, gestures, etc., as all these constantly give us indications of the mental condition we have to deal with and what tone to adopt to derive most information.

5. Test his instincts carefully and seriatim, *i.e.*, (*a*) Love of life; (*b*) Desire to procreate; (*c*) Love of offspring; (*d*) Necessity to energise; (*e*) Appetite for food and drink; (*f*) Various social instincts.

6. Test his mental faculties, his memory, power of cognition, his reasoning power, judgment, self-control, volition, etc., etc., and look out for hallucinations and delusions, depression, stupor or excitement, and altered feelings towards relatives.

7. Observe carefully his expression, articulation, writing if possible, the nutrition of the body, conformation of the head and presence of deformities in head or body.

8. Take the pulse and temperature, and examine into the condition of all the great bodily functions. Find out how he sleeps, and if he dreams and the character of the dreams. Examine into the motor and sensory functions of the brain and cord, asking about headaches and neuralgic pains.

9. Consider the case from three aspects—(*a*) *The medical* which concerns you as a physician about to treat a patient; (*b*) *the medico-legal* which concerns you and the patient as regards depriving him of his liberty and the control of his affairs, and (*c*) the *medico-psychological* which includes all the mental problems that arise from a study of the case.

10. Exclude the following conditions from the case: drunkenness, drugging, meningitis, cerebritis, syphilis, the specific fevers, sunstroke, gross brain disease, traumatic lesions, delirium tremens, the effects of moral shock or the delirium that precedes death.

11. In studying a case of insanity remember that physical and mental symptoms are common to all forms of insanity and do not look on them as due to separate entities.

12. Remember that your patient's statements can in no way be relied on, and that by your own observation, reasoning and medical examination you must distinguish between the true and the false, and find what the false is due to, whether it be with intent to deceive, or due to delusions or to deranged consciousness.

13. In some cases owing to the patient's cunning, etc., it is necessary, for his own safety or that of his relatives, for the preservation of his property, etc., etc., *to conceal your profession* and the object of your visit. One must remember, however, that relatives and others often desire that guile should be practised where there is absolutely no need for it and that deceit must not be resorted to unless when absolutely necessary.

14. Silence, obstinacy, stupidity and other negative symptoms should be noted and are valuable aids in diagnosis and treatment.

15. Compare the patient as seen by you with your mental picture of the person you have known or had described to you and note wherein the difference lies.

16. Make a blood examination where possible estimating the number of leucocytes per c.mm. and the percentages of the various types.

17. The chief problems you have to solve are :—(1) Is the patient mentally affected or not ? (2) If so, is he sufficiently affected to be regarded as irresponsible and insane ? (3) What type of insanity are you dealing with ? (4) What treatment should you adopt and what is your prognosis ? (5) What risks are there in the case ? (*a*) to the patient, (*b*) to others. (6) Can the case be safely treated at home or should it be moved to an asylum ? (7) If treated at home, can reliable attendance be obtained ?

18. Inform the patient's relatives and guardians of the risks attendant on the case and impress on them the extreme necessity for care and watchfulness. If there be cause for hope, let them know it, but be guarded, as our knowledge of mental diseases is by no means perfect as yet, and even the most experienced alienists make errors at times. Make the patient's relatives take their due responsibility in curtailing his liberty and sending him to an asylum. If you undertake to treat the case in a private house, do so only on condition that proper attendants are arranged for and placed under your exclusive orders.

CHAPTER VIII.

BRIEF DISCUSSION OF THE MAIN DIFFERENCES BETWEEN EUROPEAN AND INDIAN PSYCHOSES.

I. **The Influence of a Tropical Climate upon Neurotic Individuals.**—It is, I think, an established fact that neuroses and psychoses are more common among Europeans and their descendants in hot climates, and in a way the climate may be said to be an essential factor in their developement. The average European in the tropics does not alter his mode of living in any material way. He eats an abundant flesh diet, imbibes alcoholic beverages freely and displays an energy in the pursuit both of business and pleasure which is in strong contrast to the calm placidity of the native. As a result of this he sooner or later falls a victim to dyspepsia, and, when this condition becomes chronic, the subject is naturally more liable to metabolic or bacterial toxæmias and a train of nervous symptoms arise which may pursue him until death. If Europeans, however, were to conform more to the diet and customs of the natives around them such bodily and mental disturbances would be much less frequent. The same condition applies to the rising generation of Indians who, being more highly educated, have adopted to a greater or less extent many European habits and customs, and these, on constitutions unsuited to them, have much more marked results than on Europeans.

The regular recurrence too of a long maintained high temperature for practically one-half of the year, accompanied as it is for the latter three months by excessive atmospheric humidity, tells heavily on people accustomed to a more temperate and drier climate, for constant heat combined with constant humidity is extremely hard to bear and lucky indeed is the man who emerges from the ordeal unscathed. The most common result of these is an intractable insomnia, to which in time is superadded physical and mental lethargy and an inconquerable disinclination both for physical as well as for mental exertion. All energy is lost, the man's mental faculties become dulled, irritability and depression follow on, and finally there is an ever-increasing excitability culminating at times in explosions of open violence. As a rule maniacal conditions are more common than states of depression in such conditions and are probably largely due to the abuse of alcohol and quinine so commonly seen in the tropics.

II. **Psychoses peculiar to India.**—The large majority of mental diseases are common to both Eastern and Western races and only a few, in fact very few, forms of insanity exist which can be said to be peculiar to India. The abuse of preparations of Indian hemp, and opium is much more prevalent among Asiatics than Europeans, especially the abuse of Indian hemp, and mental symptoms due to this cause alone form a very large percentage of the admissions into Indian asylums. "Running amuck" as it is called in Northern India, or "amok" as it is termed in the Southern part of the peninsula, is almost invariably due to an excessive indulgence in *Cannabis indica*. The patient, as a rule, broods over some fancied wrong or slight until life becomes unbearable, and he determines to end it. With this object in view he has recourse to drugs, with the object of inducing a state of frenzy, and in most cases Cannabis indica is the one chosen. When absolutely beside himself with the effect of the poison he seizes his weapon and rushes blindly forth, cutting and hacking at every one he sees, killing and maiming all he meets until a timely bullet or sword cut puts an end to the slaughter by causing his death.

As cretinism is endemic in some villages in Switzerland, so we have in the Punjab a comparatively large number of microcephalic imbeciles of comparatively uniform type and commonly known as "Shah Daula's mice." The term "mice" is applied to them owing to the conformation of the cranium, which with the flattened skulls and prominent ears gives them a certain amount of resemblance to these animals, and the rest of the name is obtained from the tomb or shrine of a saint of that name in Gujrat, under whose protection they are supposed to be.

Until late years the priests in charge of this shrine used to hire them out to *faquirs* and *yogis*, who took them round the country begging; but this has now practically been put a stop to owing to the frequent and brutal ill-treatment which they met with as a rule at the hands of their masters. They are all well under average stature, but except for the microcephalic head and outstanding ears show no marked deformity otherwise. A large percentage of them appear, however, to be deaf and dumb, and strabismus is common among them, indicating probably some error in refraction or other visual defect. They are capable of being taught simple employments, and are by no means immodest or indecent, and as a rule show none of the revolting tendencies or depraved appetites so commonly seen among other types of imbeciles. Nothing is known as to how they originate, in most cases no hereditary influence being traceable, and a "chuha" may often be found with absolutely normal parents and three or four healthy brothers and sisters. They apparently are almost, if not quite, all sprung from the lowest classes. It is possible they are due to the custom, prevalent in those parts, of childless women going to pray and vow a dedication to the shrine if their prayers are heard and they are blessed with a child. Not that I fancy mental influence has anything to do with it, but, as the women stay there for several days, it is quite possible that the guardians of the shrine every now and then have recourse to one of the male microcephalics to ensure that some of the childless women who spend the night at the shrine may reproduce a "chuha," and so maintain the reputation of the tomb.

It is a common belief that this condition is due to pressure exerted in infancy by means of iron caps, but there is no confirmative evidence of this so far as I know, any *post-mortems* which have been done showing apparently normal bones, except for the contractions in every diameter of the skull.

III. **Differences of Incidence and Manifestations of Psychoses common to both the East and the West.**—Owing to differences in habits, customs and temperament the evidences of insanity among Indians vary greatly from what one looks for among Europeans. Thus, if an ordinary native woman of Northern India voluntarily appeared in public with her head uncovered, one would consider it strong presumptive evidence of mental derangement, though one would think nothing of a European woman doing so. In the same way if a European behaved as so many *faquirs* do, he would probably be promptly seized and put in an asylum, while a native can act in this way and nothing is thought about it. Innumerable other examples of this sort, arising from differences in habits, customs, environments and temperaments, can be quoted.

The differences in the laws, in Great Britain and India, too, affect very greatly the types of insanity met with in asylums in these two countries. Thus, in India owing to the wording of the law only those insanes who are too dangerous and troublesome to be left in their relatives' charge, or who are found wandering about helpless and unprotected are placed in asylums.* The people of India, too, have an innate objection to sending their sick relatives away from home. The result of these two causes is, that the numbers of insane under asylum treatment in India form an infinitesimal percentage of the

---

* Act IV of 1912 has considerably altered this state of matters, and it is possible that in a short time many more cases may be voluntarily brought to asylums for treatment, under the terms this Act, than has been the case under the old legislation.

whole population. Also if we set aside those cases suffering from secondary dementia after acute insanity, the remainder may be compared as a whole to a collection of all the most violent and destructive patients from British asylums. The natural tendency of the insane to revert to their original type of mentalisation undoubtedly has some effect in producing this result also, and explains to a certain extent the relative excess in the incidence of mania over that of melancholia, and the comparative rarity of suicidal attempts while homicidal outbursts are so frequently seen.

Custom is, I think, mainly responsible for the disgusting way so many insanes in asylums in India besmear themselves, and indeed anything else they can reach, with excreta, for the habit of "leeping" their houses and the primitive sanitary arrangements so common in villages is not conducive to any very high standard of cleanliness. Here, however, one must remember that sanitary arrangements in asylums in India differ greatly from those prevailing in Great Britain, and as a result there is more opportunity for uncleanliness in the former case. The religious beliefs and caste prejudices too largely affect not only the symptoms, but the whole course of treatment in India.

Judging by asylum admissions as a whole one would therefore be inclined to say that insanity is much less frequent and as a rule of a more violent, more maniacal, more incurable type in India. When, however, we remember the points discussed above and consider that melancholics are, on the whole, quite amenable to treatment at home, and if we also note the comparatively large percentages of katatonia, hebephrenia and paranoia, cases which are universally admitted to be sprung from neurotic stock. Then, I think, one can but come to one conclusion, *viz.* :—that insanity is at least as rife in India as in Britain, if not more so, and that probably, if every case of insanity treated outside asylums were noted, the relative percentages of melancholia and mania would be materially altered and approximate much more closely to European figures than is the case with our present statistics. In other words, though the class of cases met with in asylums in India is on the whole more maniacal than those seen in English asylums, yet, taking into account the considerations noted above, the probability is, that there is really much less difference in type than would at first appear to be the case ; also though from asylum statistics insanity seems much less rife in India than in England, it is probable that if every case of mental disease were reported, as is done in England, it would be found that insanity is fully as rife if not more so, in India.

PART II.

CHAPTER IX.

NEURASTHENIC AND HYSTERICAL CONDITIONS.

STRICTLY speaking these conditions do not fall under the head of insanity, but the border line between such sufferers and the insane is so ill-defined, and these conditions often prove such a source of confusion to the ordinary practitioner, that I think it as well to discuss them briefly before entering upon a description of the various types of insanity.

I. NEURASTHENIA.

Definition.—Neurasthenia may be defined roughly as a nervous condition affecting as a rule those of a well marked neurotic heredity, who, though they escape insanity, still show a well marked train of symptoms, both mental and physical, which generally affects the sufferers throughout their entire life.

Ætiology.—*A tainted heredity* is undoubtedly the most common predisposing cause of this affection, though in many instances the disease might never have occurred had it not been for the chance occurrence of some illness or trouble, which caused primarily instability of the nervous centres, and later a derangement of the metabolism of the whole of the organism. *Exhausting processes*, such as overstudy, prolonged lactation, pregnancy and sexual excesses; *the result of severe illness; chronic intoxication from drugs* as alcohol and carbon disulphide; *sudden shock and long continued mental strain, etc., etc.,* are all possible exciting causes of neurasthenia, whether combined with a neurotic heredity or by themselves. The large variety of possible causes of the malady shows one that each case should be carefully studied from an ætiological point of view and its treatment carried out on this basis, for it is obvious that treatment, producing good results in a case of neurasthenia resulting, say, from a railway accident, is by no means the treatment one would adopt for a case due to chronic alcoholism.

Symptomatology.—Numerous as are the causes of this condition still more so are the symptoms to which it gives rise, and every new case furnishes to a careful observer yet another combination to add to the multitude already accumulated. There are, however, in nearly every case certain prominent and fairly constant physical symptoms which may be picked out as characteristic of the condition. Among such may be noted *neuro-muscular asthenia, insomnia, mental depression, headache, pains in the back, cardiac disturbances* and *dyspeptic troubles.*

Neuro-muscular asthenia.—This is universally admitted to be the most frequent objective sign of the disease. The patient is always tired, the slightest exertion, whether physical or mental, seeming to cause an overwhelming fatigue, and as a result practically the whole day is spent on a lounge or easy chair. An examination of the muscles of such a patient shows that, though flaccid perhaps, they are still capable of considerable energy and the dynamometer at first shows no great diminution of muscular power. After the tests have been repeated several times, however, the muscles are found to have lost part of their power, so that apparently the condition is one more of mental than physical impotence. True paralysis or contractures never co-exist with neurasthenia, the patient being capable of executing any ordinary co-ordinate movement, but there seems an incapacity to store up dynamic force enough for prolonged exertion. The tendon reflexes if tested are found absolutely normal in neurasthenia pure and simple, and if there be any increase or diminution in these then the presence of some organic disease complicating the neurasthenia must be looked for. All degrees and varieties of this neuro-muscular asthenia are met with, from a mere physical and mental lassitude in the morning, which passes off as the day advances, allowing the patient to take some pleasure and interest in his duties and surroundings, to actual confinement to bed. As a rule the diminution of the cardiac force and the relaxation of the arteries are at their acme in the early morning, and as the day proceeds and the vessels become filled by the products of digestion, the vascular tone increases and accounts for the accession of nervous energy as the day advances.

Insomnia.—This is the most troublesome symptom of neurasthenia with which we have to deal, also the most unyielding to treatment. It is largely due to the gastro-intestinal disturbances present, though undoubtedly lack of muscular exertion, cardiac irregularities and diminished vascular tone also participate in its production. It occurs in a variety of forms, thus the patient may fall asleep soon after retiring only to wake after two or three hours and toss about till morning when he arises tired and unrefreshed. In other cases sleep does not come readily, the patient lies awake listening to the irregular tumult of his heart, obsessions disturb his tranquility, formication, twitchings or contractures drive away the longed-for sleep just as it seems within his grasp, and only towards morning does sleep overtake him and give him two or three hours of the longed-for rest. It is remarkable how slight the evil effects of this insomnia seem to be, and one is often inclined to believe, on this account, that the patient's account is either wilfully or unintentionally false, but in all such cases a little watching will prove the truth of the statement. Few neurasthenics show much inclination to sleep in the day time, but occasionally a case may be met with where, with the nocturnal insomnia, there is irresistible drowsiness during the day. Even the little sleep which is obtained is by no means restful or refreshing. Terrible and appalling dreams disturb repose, and time and again the sufferer wakes, terrified and soaked in perspiration, from some terrifying vision. These visions arise from the anxious mind with which such cases seek repose, the mental processes being carried on in imperfect form when consciousness is partially lost.

Mental Depression.—One of the earliest symptoms of neurasthenia, especially when the condition is due to prolonged mental strain, is loss of memory and inability to recall events. Names of people go beyond recall, writing and conversation are cut short for want of words, books and papers are read without any recollection of their contents remaining and the details of business fall into entire abeyance. The power of looking after oneself and one's business vanishes and the whole attention remaining is concentrated upon the unfortunate and helpless condition one has fallen into. Such conditions are especially common in cases of an hereditary type and are more frequently seen in women than in men, and, as with all neurasthenic conditions, they are more marked in the morning tending to pass off in the afternoon.

Headache.—About the onset of puberty those with a tendency to neurasthenia begin to show the first signs of instability in paroxysmal attacks of "sick headache." Girls, as a rule, suffer about the time of the menstrual periods and with males too the attacks seem to come on with similar regularity, probably owing to the regular rise and fall already noted as occurring in the blood-pressure.

The headache of neurasthenia is characteristic and present in greater or less degree in practically every case. It may be continuous over months or even years though at times it is intermittent. Physical and mental exertion invariably increase it, and, as with so many other neurasthenic symptoms, it is always worst in the morning, tending to pass off during the day.

Painful sensation is as a rule absent or only slight in amount, the patient complaining of a feeling of weight or constriction around the temples. Slight vertigo, roaring in the ear, retinal hyperæsthesias and muscæ volitantes and other phenomena accompany it. The headache is not diffuse in all cases but may be localised to certain areas, the most favourite site being the occipital and nuchial regions and here actual pain is complained of much more frequently than in any other region.

Pains in the Back.—This symptom of neurasthenia is very much more commonly seen in women than in men, and any attempt at motion suffices to bring it out. It is aggravated by the occurrence of the menstrual periods, the pains and aches being materially increased by the congestion of the organs of generation, and ovarian neuralgias are its common accompaniment. In men it is frequently confounded with rheumatoid or prea-taxic pains, and often gives rise to mental depression or hypochondriasis.

Accompanying the pains various hyperæsthesias of the genital organs, formication and other derangements of sensation are met with.

Cardiac Disturbances.—An irregular and tumultuous action is the most common of these and is probably due to a transient inhibition of the vagus fibres (Lehre), which probably arises from the weakness of the reflex centres peculiar to neurasthenia. The immediate cause is probably in most cases fright or anxiety, though probably sexual excesses, alcoholism and mental strain contribute in producing it. In one type of case the rhythm is regular and not perceptibly above the normal, but the arterial tension is increased, giving rise to the various other symptoms so commonly seen in neurasthenics. In such conditions slight emotion may bring on a high degree of irregularity with anxiety and præcordial distress, such attacks lasting for a few minutes and leaving the patient as a rule much exhausted. In other cases the cardiac rate is increased sometimes up to 130 per minute and there is a diminution in arterial tension. When a nervous seizure occurs in such cases the pulse becomes small, the tension is markedly diminished and the pulse rate is increased by twenty-five to thirty beats. Accompanying this there is extreme reflex irritability and a feeling of great lassitude and fatigue ; and at times vertigo, trembling and even unconsciousness may accompany the attack, which may last from a few minutes up to five or six hours. Warm baths with cold applications over the cardiac region, and the exhibition of alcohol and the bromides combined with aconite are indicated during the acute attack and between attacks full nourishing diet, tonics, malt liquors, etc., should be made full use of.

Digestive Troubles.—These are practically an invariable accompaniment of all neurasthenic conditions, but their character and degree varies greatly with individual cases. In by far the majority of cases it appears as a gastro-intestinal disturbance, atonic in character. In mild cases there is not much reduction in weight, abdominal discomfort being the main subjective symptom, but in the more severe cases loss of weight is often very marked, and it is a common cause of the anæmia so prevalent among neurasthenics.

In such cases, as a rule, after the ingestion of food there is an immediate sensation of comfort and well being, which, however, is soon replaced by vague feelings of weight and distention in the gastric region and frequent eructations of gas. After the food has passed from the stomach to the intestine the gaseous fermentation is partially arrested and some relief is experienced for a time, but the intestinal contents soon become fermented too and borborygmi begin, which may be so severe as to cause a sensitive patient to seek solitude and shun all company. Severe colic often accompanies this stage and may be a great trial, lasting for an hour or more until expulsion of the gas per rectum brings gradual relief and the patient returns to his usual condition. Such symptoms, as a rule, follow after every meal and utterly prevent the patient from having any pleasure in life, though they rarely produce any marked emaciation. The cause of this atonic dyspepsia is the subacidity of the gastric juices, as shown by the phloroglucinol phenylin and other tests, this subacidity allowing fermentation to proceed which the presence of ·3% of acid is quite sufficient to check for a long time. The fermentation is probably started by micro-organisms which, having collected between the teeth, get mixed with the food during the process of mastication and thus get carried with it into the stomach where the absence of hydrochloric acid allows fermentation to begin, and this is still further increased by the alkaline juices of the duodenum.

Constipation nearly always accompanies nervous dyspepsia in all its forms, and when the bowels are moved by purgatives or enemata the fæces are expelled as hard scyballous masses. When there is chronic catarrhal affection of the small intestine, as sometimes happens, diarrhœa may replace the constipation and much emaciation occurs, though as a rule life is rarely threatened. In most neurasthenic cases the tone of the muscles of the alimentary canal is fairly well maintained and in consequence dilatation of the stomach is but rarely seen, the ingesta passing through at a fairly normal rate.

The dyspepsia from subacidity is most unyielding to treatment and may continue for years without amelioration, though, as a rule, the exhibition of acids lessens the fermentation, renders the patient more comfortable and promotes nutrition.

It is often extremely difficult to differentiate more severe cases from some gastric tumour. In both instances the hydrochloric acid of the gastric juice is diminished or absent, and the emaciation, the yellow, dried up skin, the markedly progressive deterioration of the blood is also common to both types of disease. The absence of a tumour in the gastric region and the history of suffering from various other cardinal symptoms of neurasthenia for some months, are the main points which help us in our differential diagnosis.

Nervous diarrhœas are often seen in neurotic people, and often the mere thought of a railway journey or some public ordeal is sufficient to start an attack which ceases so soon as the cause is over.

The Mental Symptoms of Neurasthenics are much more difficult to comprehend and elicit than the physical ones, and are by no means invariably present, though in a large proportion of cases a careful and tactful enquiry may bring them to light. These mental phenomena are extremely varied in character, but as a rule, arise from obsessions or imperative ideas and from these are evolved states of mixed motor-emotional agitation.

From the imperfect adjustment of the brain equipoise, whether in the alert or subconscious state, certain dominant ideas obtrude themselves and, owing to the imperfect volition of the patient, assert and reassert themselves at all times, gaining a morbid clearness which impresses them so on the mind of the patient that, unless some change of habits or surroundings intervenes, the patient's whole life is influenced by them. These imperative conceptions are recognised by the patient as absurd, but to resist them only produces mental distress, while yielding to them only increases their power over the unhappy individual, and in either case his condition is almost unbearable. They are palpably in no way connected with hallucinations, and being recognised as false by the patient cannot be classed as delusions.

Motor-Mental Agitation.—The obsession forcing a patient to some foolish or revolting act often brings on such a state of agitation that incessant motion can alone relieve it. In such circumstances the patient walks about his room, wringing his hands, and weeping and praying in an indescribable state of mental hyperæsthesia until gradually a sense of relief is experienced and he becomes again calm and collected. These attacks resemble greatly the exacerbations seen so often in acute mania and excited melancholia, but are much more transient and less intense.

Neurasthenic Anxiety and Compulsory Ideas.—These, as with the majority of the mental symptoms of neurasthenia, are as a rule due to a loss or diminution of the power of volition. They arise usually either as a result of half-conscious dream states giving rise to a form of auto-suggestion, or from long continued habits which gradually gain more and more dominance until finally they affect the whole life of the patient. As a rule, the patients recognise their absurdity, and at times even make feeble attempts to overcome them, but their volition is too weak to sustain the struggle long and they soon return to their former condition of terror and anxiety. These obsessions therefore are markedly different from those of the paranoiac who is convinced of the truth of his delusions, but, at the same time, the constant presence of one train of thought has an undoubted effect upon unstable brain matter and occasionally assumes pathological proportions.

The imperative ideas of the anxious neurasthenic may assume an infinite variety of form. Some may arise from perfectly natural aversions such as the dread of filth, of poison, of infection, of solitude, etc. To many such forms distinctive names have been given, *e.g.*, *agoraphobia*, the fear of open spaces; *claustrophobia*, the fear of being in a closed room; *zoophobia*, the fear of animals, etc.

The "*delire de toucher et de doute*" of some authors is simply one form of this affection. In the first the sufferer has an irresistible desire to touch a certain type of article, thus for example he may have an intense desire to read every piece of writing he comes across, torn scraps picked up in the road or from a sweeper's basket, private documents on an official's desk, it is all the same to him, read them he must and does, and naturally he is constantly in hot water. The reverse of this is frequently seen, thus there is a marked antipathy to touch certain articles and forced contact arouses a lively disquietude which can only be assuaged by repeated ablutions.

The "folie de doute" is a condition where every object and action is a cause of interminable arguing and reasoning, and often renders the sufferer unfit to continue his work owing to the apprehensions that some error may arise which might have a serious effect upon his career.

As a rule neurasthenic symptoms show a tendency to be intermittent in character, and the majority of cases show a tendency to temporarily improve in the hotter seasons and recrudesce during the colder months, owing to the effects of vasomotor paresis being less marked during the hotter seasons.

Diagnosis.—As can be readily understood, it is often a matter of great difficulty to distinguish neurasthenia from *incipient general paralysis of the insane, cerebral syphilis, tabes dorsalis* and various other forms of organic cerebral and spinal disease, especially if a distinct history of venereal disease be obtainable. One has also to distinguish it from various types of insanity. In each case one must go carefully into the history of the patient and the mode of onset of the illness, asking especially about the symptoms, both physical and mental, detailed above. Next a careful examination of all deep and superficial reflexes must be made, and signs of paralysis or contractures looked for. Having ascertained all these fully and carefully one has then to go over the notes made during the examination and estimate to the best of one's power the condition present and, if the cardinal symptoms and conditions above noted be kept in mind, a fairly correct diagnosis will sooner or later be arrived at.

Treatment.—This is invariably a matter of much difficulty in neurasthenics. Every case must be carefully considered on its own merits and the treatment based on this, for what may prove beneficial in one case may be useless or worse than useless in many others. Each case must, therefore, be studied carefully by itself, careful enquiry made as to any hereditary taint and the presence of acute diseases during the earlier years of life, as to the possibility of the symptoms having been aggravated by excessive venery, and indulgence in alcoholism or masturbation, and whether there be indications of secret indulgence in any drugs.

All these having been carefully enquired into, the treatment divides itself into four heads, *hygienic, dietetic, moral* and *medicinal.* Weir Mitchell's treatment is based on the first three of these heads.

Hygienic.—The sanitation of the patient's surroundings should be carefully looked to as regards drainage, ventilation and lighting. The water-supply should be looked to, and examined both chemically and bacteriologically and proper bathing should be insisted on, careful instructions being given as to the time and temperature of the baths. Some neurasthenics improve wonderfully with cold baths and douches in the morning, while with others cold bathing does more harm than good and lukewarm or even hot baths are required, and in such cases night time as a rule is the best time for bathing as it calms obsessions and has good results in promoting sleep.

Climate, too, has to be considered, and, as a rule, it will be found that excitable, emotional cases do best at fairly high altitudes, while depressed cases with slow, imperfect digestion are better at lower levels. Removal from all business cares and change of scene to a free life in the country, from the hot monotonous existence of a town or cantonment in the plains to the bracing air and lovely scenery of some quiet hill station, often works wonders in the restitution of a broken down nervous system. Removal from his own family circle to the society of strangers in some bracing quiet place, where there is, however, distraction sufficient to prevent brooding, is what we should aim at, as well as regulating the patient's life so that every hour of the day may have something to stimulate his flagging energies and give him an interest in life.

Dietetic.—By far the majority of neurasthenics are anæmic and run down and really require what we may call a surplus of food, and it is a mistake to think that because dyspepsia is present food should be exhibited only at long intervals. It is true that in a certain number of cases with slow digestions three meals a day have excellent results, but as a rule it will be found better in all neurasthenic cases to remove them from their previous diet and feed them on "slops" for a time, adding gradually one food-stuff after another, until we find what is most suitable for our patient and gives the best results.

Milk, eggs, a moderate amount of meat, both red and white, fish, vegetables especially cabbages, carrots and those rich in chlorophyl may all be added gradually to the diet, but potatoes as a rule are best avoided. Fruit can be given fairly freely and especially so if cooked. The imbibing of fluids should be carefully regulated and only a limited amount allowed at meals as otherwise indigestion is almost sure to result. A useful means of quieting the patient and inducing sleep will be found in the administration of some hot broth, milk or cocoa just at bedtime, though it may not answer in all cases.

Moral.—The influence the physician, by unfailing tact, care and sympathy, is able to obtain over the patient, is of invaluable aid in his treatment of the case. Only too often is the condition of the patient made worse by his relatives and friends misunderstanding the state of affairs and deriding his depression and feeble will power. This as a rule far from stimulating him to fresh efforts at self-control only makes him still more miserable, and he sinks farther and farther into the depths of despair. A little sympathy and kindliness combined with the requisite firmness in carrying out the treatment laid down, is what is required, and our efforts should be directed to attain this end, and, though exhibiting the necessary sympathy, yet avoid a leniency which by extending too far might equally militate against the results we aim at.

Hypnotic suggestion has been advised by many Continental authorities, but experience has shown it to be more harmful than beneficial as it tends to still further weaken the already deficient will power. All that should be attempted in this line is, to impress on the slack attention of the patient by well considered words and actions that he is by no means incurable and his malady is purely a functional one, the cure of which rests largely in his own hands. The pathogenesis of the "phobias" and other imperative conceptions should always be carefully explained to intelligent patients and their aid sought in overcoming them.

In many cases of the severer types it is absolutely necessary to take the patients away from their surroundings and place them under the care of a nurse who, under proper medical supervision, has complete control of the case. The Weir Mitchell treatment consists of this combined with massage, electricity and over-feeding. Complete isolation is only necessary in a few cases and in the large majority rest, massage and dieting make up the essentials of our treatment. The mental qualities of the nurse should be carefully ascertained before any arrangements are made, for a firm but sympathetic nature is essential to the cure of such cases.

Therapeutic measures.—The exhibition of medicines is not so much required in this condition as the prevention of the patient lavishing money on endless quack medicines and imbibing them, probably with disastrous results to himself. Any new advertisement seen or drug mentioned by friends sends the patient flying to the chemist to purchase it, and many thus become addicted to some drug habit or alcoholic indulgence which is often much more difficult to overcome than the primary trouble.

Neurasthenia being essentially due to lack of a reserve of nervous energy, rest in bed is an absolute necessity in all cases for a few days at least. When by this means a certain modicum of energy has been stored up, carefully regulated walking or driving may be indulged in. With a certain number of chronic cases, however, too prolonged a rest is harmful, and they should be gently forced to take interest in what is going on around them and be roused from their self absorption. Massage and electricity are often excellent adjuvants during the period of enforced rest, though at times, and in certain cases, they seem to have a debilitating effect and are therefore contraindicated.

Hydrotherapy.—As already noted carefully regulated baths are often of the utmost service in treating such conditions. Extremes of temperature and too prolonged immersion are always to be avoided. Wrapping the body in a wet sheet for from 15 to 30 minutes has often most beneficial effects, especially if it be followed by a brisk rubdown with a coarse towel. The temperature for this should be 85°—90°F. as a start, the water being gradually cooled or heated as the patient's condition requires. Cold douches and very hot plunge baths are to be avoided, though a tepid plunge at bedtime is often most useful in inducing sleep.

Drugs.—All neurasthenic cases require some tissue building tonic owing to their state of extreme physical weakness. In addition to this some harmless sedative as tincture of valerian, paraldehyde, or trional may be given to quiet the patient and prevent his sending to the chemist for all sorts of quack medicines for one and all of his fancied ailments.

The most useful forms of iron are the peptonates of iron and manganese or the subcarbonate of iron especially in combination with other drugs, as is the case with several tabloids and capsules prepared by Messrs. Burroughs Wellcome & Co.

Preparations of phosphates are useful adjuvants, perhaps the most useful being the glycerophosphates in combination with cod liver oil or somatose.

Strychnine from its general tonic effects, is good and especially so in cases of gastro-intestinal atony.

Hydrochloric acid, alone or combined with pepsin, is invaluable when fermentative dyspepsia is present.

Prognosis.—A permanent cure of neurasthenia is in all cases most problematical. A certain number improve sufficiently to enable them to take an active interest again in life but relapses are frequent. The prognosis should therefore in all cases be a guarded one, and especially so if there be any marked hereditary taint ascertainable.

NEURASTHENIC PSYCHOSES.

Mental symptoms playing such a large part in all cases of neurasthenia (and the liability to toxic absorptions in such cases being so great) it is surprising how few, among the large numbers of such cases, overstep the boundary and become insane. When such cases do occur they are, as one would naturally expect, of the melancholic type, maniacal states very rarely being seen. The attacks generally occur at the climax of an exhaustion paroxysm and quickly respond to rest, feeding and sedatives, though a certain small number with marked neurotic heredity may run on to secondary dementia.

Masturbation is a frequent cause of a more protracted form of mental confusion, amounting at times to stupor, and in such cases the prognosis is by no means hopeful.

Some cases, generally those of marked neurotic family, pass into a condition of paranoia and for such cases recovery is practically hopeless and the frequency of aural hallucinations with the resulting danger to the public renders it necessary to place such cases in asylums.

HYSTERICAL PSYCHOSES.

Though hysteria and neurasthenia are, pathogenically, practically similar conditions, both being due to an incomplete developement of the higher cortical centres concerned in mentalisation, yet, clinically, they differ widely in their manifestations, and when, as occasionally happens, the two conditions are found in one and the same individual, the diagnosis is often a matter of extreme difficulty.

The main points to look for are, in hysteria, the convulsive crises, the hemianæsthesias and segmentary anæsthesias, the contractures and paralyses, with narrowing of the field of vision and derangements of colour vision. In neurasthenia we have the constant dull headache, the motor asthenia, the rachialgia, the atonic dyspepsias, insomnia and the other symptoms arising from defective vasomotor innervation. The mental conditions of the two diseases are also wholly different. In hysteria we see a marked reaction to emotion resulting in histrionic displays, or simulation, from auto-suggestion or extrinsic suggestion, of paralyses and contractures. Defects of mental co-ordination and of the will power render it almost impossible to catch the attention of the patient, and, owing to defects of memory as well as of the moral sense, it is impossible to rely on the statement of any one suffering from hysteria. In neurasthenia again we meet with patients so self centred that they are irritable and morbidly depressed, though not so much so as to constitute a true melancholia. They are the prey of innumerable impulses and obsessions and suffer from transitory defects of memory which however can be corrected if attention be drawn to them.

The Ætiology of hysteria must undoubtedly be looked for in hereditary taint, aggravated by defective education, lack of proper control at home and indulgence in either emotional or sexual passions in early life. The greater and less repressed emotional nature of women renders them the most frequent sufferers, and indeed certain characteristics of hysteria appear to be only exaggerations of well known feminine traits.

The most common period of life for hysterical manifestations to appear is the post-pubescent age, teeming as it is with the natural longings that follow the change from incomplete to active developement of the sexual functions, and especially great are its effects upon girls, who perhaps up to that time have lived the life of a tom-boy but are then bound down by the trammels of social life, and, meeting every hour of their lives with the repression of their natural emotions, are driven to concentrate their attention upon themselves and in many cases upon those organs so lately sprung into functional being.

The deviations from normal mentalisation proper to hysteria are as a rule of a transitory character and follow after the convulsive crises with which they have a direct relation. They may be divided into two classes: (a) *Those belonging to the interparoxysmal period;* (b) *Those immediately succeeding the attack.*

(*a*) **Interparoxysmal period.**—The psychoses characteristic of this period are *amnesia, loss of will power, aboulia or loss of the faculty of attention, great emotional instability* and *excessive reaction to suggestion.* The patients may be gay, active and mischievous; or the reverse conditions may prevail and they may be passive and apathetic.

Amnesia is usually present to a greater or less extent and as already noted is one of the causes of the mendacity so common in this condition. In severe cases and after frequent attacks all remembrance of the past is lost and only recalled during the paroxysms.

The *loss of volition and faculty of attention* are found in other conditions and by themselves are not pathognomonic of an hysterical condition. It at times takes the form of a *folie de doute*, but as a rule simply incapacitates the patient from carrying on his ordinary daily duties,—not from perversity or obstinacy, but simply from sheer lack of will power. This therefore is in direct antithesis to the powerlessness arising from fixed ideas of repugnance so commonly seen in neurasthenia.

Mental hysteria, a condition where one sees all the mental but none of the physical stigmata of this condition, is common in India among Europeans, natives and especially among Eurasians. It is characterised by an extremely emotional nature which is always to be seen at work, as evidenced by capriciousness, sentimentality, irritability and great changefulness of mood. Such persons have but little self control, are morbidly nervous, and quick perhaps at chaff and repartee, lack judgment and are incapable of doing any work requiring great mental effort.

(*b*) **Post paroxysmal Psychoses.**—These are numerous and varied both in type and degree, stretching from various states of exaltation and depression through delusional conditions to somnambulism and stupor. All of these are, as a rule, transitory and but little or no remembrance of the seizure remains after recovery. Some, such as somnambulism and lethargy, are not necessarily preceded by a seizure, though a condition resembling epilepsie larvée is undoubtedly present in all such cases.

An almost constant symptom in such cases is the presence of hallucinations of sight and hearing, and I think there can be but little doubt, but that the visions ascribed to nuns and others in the past and which have given rise to many of the shrines and chapels famous now for their "faith cures" are but double examples of this, the visions in the first place being but hysterical delusions and the cures being mainly the removal by suggestion of hysterical paralyses and contractures.

In the delirium of *hystero-epilepsy* consciousness is lost, the patients at one moment shouting, singing and dancing and being restrained only with the greatest difficulty, and the next being sunk in an almost stuporose condition. With this a maniacal condition at times is seen, with an inconceivable flow of language in which, however, there is a tendency to the repetition of words and phrases which renders it unlike the logorrhœa of the true maniac.

Lethargy.—May follow a severe seizure or come on without warning, and may last from a few minutes to a few weeks in which case it is in all probability the equivalent of a seizure. Cataleptic conditions of the muscular system have been noted during such attacks and, if the condition lasts long, artificial feeding may be necessary and emaciation becomes marked.

In some cases the excitement after an hysterical attack is prolonged over an indefinite period, assuming a chronic hallucinatory type very commonly seen in many of the "exhaustion psychoses," but here the alternations of confusion and stupor with hallucinatory ecstacy, or even hysterical convulsions, are extremely characteristic.

True mania and melancholia may complicate but never arise from a case of hysteria, and though a form of paranoia after hysteria has been described by Krafft-Ebing I think most authorities at the present day are inclined to doubt its reality.

Suicide may occur in hysterical conditions and undoubtedly many attempts are made, but most of these are simply to attract attention and sympathy.

Treatment.—The treatment is practically the same as for neurasthenia, and I would refer my readers to that section rather than cumber this book with a repetition of what I have already said there.

CHAPTER X.

INSANITIES OF NON-TOXIC ORIGIN.

EXHAUSTION INSANITIES.

Ætiology.—These, as a rule, are conditions of the late adult or senile periods of life when the natural reparative powers of the body begin to fail, and with men these are practically the only periods of life in which it is seen. In women, however, the disease is often seen at much earlier age periods owing to prolonged lactation, and this is specially the case in India, where the habit prevails, certainly among the lower classes, of suckling the children for two or even three years.

Heredity, nervous diseases and a neurotic temperament are all predisposing causes, while the exciting causes are innumerable, including all conditions which exhaust the physical powers.

Symptoms—Prodromata.—The attack begins insidiously, and often for some months before distinct mental symptoms manifest themselves a falling off in physical energy, dyspepsia, constipation, anæmia, atonic conditions of the circulatory system, irritability, nervousness and insomnia have been noticed by the patient and his friends.

(*a.*) **Physical.**—On seeing such a case one is at once struck by the appearance of mal-nutrition, the pallor and unhealthy condition of the skin which has a cold clammy feeling and seems to have lost the elasticity normally appertaining to it. The eyes are dull, and the attitude and expression listless and apathetic, and form a striking picture of the mental and bodily state of the sufferer. The temperature is generally subnormal. Dyspepsia and constipation are almost invariably present, and often much persuasion is required before the patient can be got to take nourishment. Anæmia is invariably present, there being, as a rule, a deficiency in the red blood corpuscles as well as in the hæmoglobin they contain. There is never any hyperleucocytosis and as a rule the polymorph percentage is lower than normal. The cardiac action is feeble, and functional murmurs are often present in the mitral and aortic areas. Œdema of the extremities is a common symptom. The skin has a dirty sallow appearance, is cold, clammy and non-elastic to the touch, and any sudden noise may suffice to bring on profuse perspiration. The urine is practically normal in all cases, and there is no marked derangement of any of the sensory or motor functions beyond the results of the general atonic condition of the whole system.

(*b.*) *Mental.*—The mental condition is invariably one of depression and confusion, varying from comparatively slight melancholic conditions to severer forms combined with delusions of suspicion, or, in the more severe cases, to a semi-stuporose condition where the patient sits listlessly all day long in one position with a sad vacant expression and can barely be roused to answer questions. The slightest attempt at even the simplest mental effort causes intense exhaustion owing to the anergic condition of the cortical centres. Cognition of time and place is unaffected, but occasionally hallucinations of sight are met with. Delusions, though not an invariable concomitant, are often met with and generally consist of suspicions of poisoning, or torturing by "electricity", "marconigrams", and "unseen agencies," or of other people talking about or laughing at the patient. The faculty of attention is deficient as is also the power of volition. Self-control is lost and the patient is obstinate and easily irritated, either getting angry or having fits of passionate weeping at the merest trifles. Memory is good both for recent and past events. The speech is lacking in life and character and seems to be a distinct effort to the patient, but it is never incoherent. The comprehension too, of questions and statements made by other people, seems at times to be a matter of difficulty to the patient. Insomnia is present in every case and is often a source of trouble in the treatment.

Treatment.—Prolonged rest in bed is essential in all cases, and a cheerful, sympathetic but strong willed attendant is a most useful and necessary adjunct. The diet should be at first light, but ample and nourishing, milk, farinaceous foods, fish, chicken, soups, etc., being given in as large quantities as the patient can be persuaded to take. When recovery is well begun, ordinary full diet should be freely given and if possible some of the malt beverages, such as beer and stout. As regards drugs, general tonics such as iron, strychnine and the phosphates are indicated for the general condition, and for insomnia veronal, trional, sulphonal, or paraldehyde in small doses (10—15 m.) may be given, though in all cases before the exhibition of hypnotics the effects of a warm bath (95°F.) and a glass of hot milk at bedtime should be tried.

Prognosis.—This is influenced largely by the age of the patient and the cause of the exhaustion. As a rule, the younger the patient is, the better the prognosis which we can give. Cases due to prolonged lactation as a rule make a fairly rapid recovery, but cases arising from severe illness or physical and mental strain progress but slowly, and are apt to pass into a condition of mild secondary dementia.

Diagnosis.—This depends mainly on the history of the patient and of any previous physical or mental strain, such as prolonged lactation, overstudy, prolonged nursing of some near relative or some severe illness. The extreme physical exhaustion and the absence of any symptoms of toxæmia are the main symptoms we have to help us in this condition.

INSANITY RESULTING FROM GROSS BRAIN LESIONS.

The brain lesions most apt to be followed by mental symptoms are those affecting the motor areas of the cortex, especially those of the left frontal lobe which implicate Broca's convolution, and, as a rule, they are of vascular origin. The mental symptoms may follow immediately after the lesion, as is almost invariably the case when aphasia is present, or they may be delayed for some months. The early symptoms are invariably of a maniacal type and may be very acute ; they are due partly to cerebral irritation from extravasated blood, partly to derangements in the nutrition of the cortex and partly perhaps to absorption of products produced by the breaking down of the effused blood corpuscles. The acute symptoms rarely last more than a few days and are followed by a condition of irritable dementia. In some cases the first acute stage may be absent and the childishness, emotionalism, extreme irritability and causeless outbursts of rage characteristic of the second stage may come on gradually. Except for paralyses according to the areas affected there are no physical symptoms worthy of note in these conditions.

Lesions of the brain have been cited at one time or another as the cause of all sorts of brain disease, such as mania and melancholia, but in by far the greater number, if not all, of such cases the probability is that no attempt has been made to exclude the possibility of a toxæmic origin for these conditions.

Epilepsy undoubtedly does follow after brain injuries, and, as a result of the cortical irritation and epileptic discharges, one finds extreme irritability and impulsiveness in such cases, and on such brains alcohol has most deleterious results, producing attacks of wild mania which often end in brutal and revolting crimes. After repeated fits one at times sees a sort of stuporose condition with loss of memory and a blunting of all the mental faculties, a sort of secondary dementia in fact.

TRAUMATIC INSANITY.

The insanity following injuries to the head is a subject of moment not only from a medical but from a medico-legal point of view, especially in so far as it concerns insurance companies, and large employers of labour, railway companies, etc., etc. Many of the traumatic neuroses are purely nervous, and many of them very obscure nervous complaints, and such cases are apt to be misinterpreted and looked on either as mere foolish fancies, or else construed as pure fiction and an attempt to obtain compensation by fraudulent means. The full comprehension of such cases is therefore a matter of importance to all medical men as without it they may unwittingly do a man gross injustice, and moreover quite possibly place themselves in an exceedingly awkward predicament.

Ætiology.—The apparent injury to the head may be only slight, or, as occurs in many cases, not a trace of injury may be found, a severe fall on the feet or gluteal region having perhaps caused a concussion of the base of the brain, quite sufficient to account for the mental symptoms but leaving no subsequent trace, or even a severe fright may suffice in cases of hereditary taint. In many cases indeed absolutely no organic basis can be found to account for the condition, and most modern authorities are agreed as to the possibility of a psychical origin for such conditions. In such cases the mental condition may be apparent at once or it may be delayed for some months, though even in these latter cases careful observation would probably reveal some slight change in character or mentalisation immediately after the incident. It is these cases, where the appearance of the symptoms is delayed, which form the great stumbling-block for the unwary and against them I would earnestly warn my readers. In such cases, where there is an interval of apparent recovery between the results of the accident and the appearance of mental symptoms, the explanation is that the recovery is only from the urgent and acute symptoms and that the later ones are of slow developement. Moreover, the recovery is rarely complete, and careful observation usually reveals one or more signs of deranged mentalisation, chief among which insomnia may be noted. Alcoholics and syphilitics are especially liable to bad effects from head injuries caused by blows or falls, and in the latter type a cranial injury may very soon be followed by general paralysis, though the injury is only a determining and not a primary cause in such cases.

Sunstroke too must be included under this head, for the neuroses following on an attack of the sun are, to all intents and purposes, such as are met with as the result of blows and falls, as, for instance, cases where after head injuries or sunstroke the patient cannot take any alcoholic beverage without revealing marked temporary mental aberration, at times even approaching an attack of maniacal frenzy.

Physical symptoms.—These naturally are mainly subjective. Headache is the most prominent and may be almost continual, though in other cases it is confined mainly to times of work or when any prolonged effort of attention is required. Defects of vision are frequently seen, the patient complaining of diplopia or of the "letters all running together" when he is reading. Noises in the ears are frequent and may be a source of much annoyance to the patient. Derangements of sensation are often present, and the patient complains often of pain in the back of the neck or in the lumbar or dorsal regions. Fine tremors may be present in the tongue, face and fingers, and bladder troubles are frequently seen owing to some indefinite complication of the innervation of the involuntary muscle. Appetite is poor, and, as a rule, chronic dyspepsia is present in most cases, leading to general ill-health and emaciation.

Mental symptoms.—These may either appear directly after the accident or may develope slowly as the acute symptoms fade away, being delayed often for weeks or months. The patient becomes very irritable and querulous and is always complaining and finding fault. He is readily fatigued by even the slightest physical or mental exertion. Memory is distinctly impaired, as is also his power of attention, and in some cases there is constant confusion and total inability to understand any communication whether written or verbal. As a result of this depression is often seen, and even attempts at suicide may be made on account of this inability to work, and the feeling that he is a burden on all his relatives or friends. Insomnia is frequent in all such cases and obsessions are often present. Many such cases too are hypochondriacal and imagine they suffer from various forms of disease as a result of the accident.

The course of such cases is usually a long one, weeks and months often passing with little or no apparent improvement taking place. In favourable cases the powers of attention and thought gradually return and the bodily condition improves, while the continual sense of fatigue disappears, memory becomes more accurate and by degrees the patient returns to his normal condition.

Diagnosis.—What is here mainly required of us is not so much to distinguish this condition from various others, such as neurasthenia or hysteria, as ability to detect the malingerer. Insurance companies and employers of labour often ask our advice regarding claims for compensation, and we must remember that, though every care should be taken to frustrate the swindler, in doing so we must do all in our power to prevent injustice to honest men. It is the whole statement of the case on which we must rely for this and not on one or two details, for the malingerer, as a rule, overacts his part and his statement of his symptoms teems with incongruities. See the patient and his friends separately and note whether their statements agree, enquiring for the presence of unlikely symptoms, as by this means the malingerer is frequently induced to betray himself. Never show any surprise at any statement or answer received, but let the patient tell his own story first, avoiding leading questions, and remember that the patient may lay particular stress on certain points which seem to him of importance, and other mental and physical changes may be gathered from his friends.

Prognosis.—This disorder is invariably a severe test of the prognostic powers of the medical attendant. Not only the severity of the accident, but the past and present history also of the patient have to be taken into consideration, and every detail carefully weighed. Two judgments are invariably required of us—(*a*) What is the immediate prospect? (*b*) What is the ultimate prognosis?

In some cases complete recovery may take place after some months or even years, while in others again there may be complete incapacity for work and earning a livelihood, though the capability of enjoying life is recovered so long as they are free from work. These are the cases which are the cause of most litigation, because the lay mind wholly fails to understand the utter incapacity there is in such cases of fixing the attention for more than a moment at a time. Each case must therefore be carefully studied on its own merits, and it must be remembered that the power of concentrating the attention, the functions of memory, volition and the like may all suffer and yet the grosser functions may remain undamaged.

Treatment.—In all cases complete cessation of work and all business matters must be insisted on, and in many cases complete rest in bed for some weeks will be found most beneficial. Baths, massage and gentle exercise are often of the utmost benefit. Diet should be of a full and nourishing nature, meals being frequent (every two hours or so) and of small amount, and nourishment should be given through the night. Severer cases require treatment in some hospital and complete removal from their friends is indicated. When convalescence is well advanced some light employment must be attempted, but fatigue must always be avoided, and it must be remembered that we should never attempt to hasten recovery, and that too early attempts to work only cause a relapse and are therefore worse than useless.

INSANITY RESULTING FROM BRAIN ANÆMIA.

Mental symptoms accompanying the constriction or occlusion of the cerebral arteries, arising from various diseases, may of course be due to the direct action on the cerebral tissue of the irritant or toxine which is the cause of the vascular lesion. It is, however, only reasonable to suppose that, apart from these conditions which will be described later, the anæmia of the cerebral cortex resulting from such constriction or occlusion of the arterial supply, is in itself sufficient to cause mental symptoms in many cases. In fact, such conditions are to be seen in every asylum, and there are certain characteristics fairly common to the group which enables us to distinguish them fairly readily.

Ætiology.—A neurotic heredity is traceable in the majority of such cases and the exciting cause is naturally the blocking of the arteries causing the brain anæmia, this blocking being due to various causes such as syphilis, gout, etc.

Symptoms.—The condition generally begins gradually and partakes of the character of a gradually increasing failure of the mental powers which imperceptibly proceeds to a complete dementia.

Physical symptoms.—The heart's action is unaffected, the rhythm being normal both as regards rate and regularity. The arterial tension in such cases is however invariably increased. There is no hyperleucocytosis present and the percentage of the various types of leucocytes remains about the normal. In fact, increased arterial tension is almost the only cardinal physical symptom in such cases, though at times various forms of paralysis are seen.

Mental symptoms.—These consist of a gradually increasing dementia with progressive loss of intelligence and capacity for work. Combined with this delusions of suspicion and unseen agency are often seen, and disorders of common sensibility are frequent, and indeed are often the cause of many of the delusions, formication being interpreted as being due to electrical agencies employed by enemies to make life unendurable.

Treatment.—Treatment in such cases should aim at removing the cause of the anæmia as far as possible and building up the general health by tonics and well-regulated exercises.

INSANITY RESULTING FROM DEPRIVATION OF THE SPECIAL SENSES.

Of the five special senses sight and hearing are, by their deprivation, undoubtedly most important in the production of psychoses. By these two senses we adapt ourselves to our surroundings and the constantly changing conditions under which we live and work, and the loss of sight or hearing places us at once at a disadvantage with our fellows. Thus it is not surprising that in persons of neurotic taint the loss of either of these senses is followed very frequently by mental symptoms.

The man who has lost the sense of sight loses his sense of position and the true knowledge of what is happening around him, and experiences a sensation of absolute helplessness which he endeavours to remove by straining all his remaining faculties to the utmost. Similarly, the man who has lost his power of hearing is deprived of sensory stimuli necessary for healthy mentalisation, and is constantly endeavouring, by means of his remaining senses, to understand what is being said around him. Under these conditions the faculties which remain are excited to excessive activity and the brain receives an over-stimulation from these senses and suffers from a deprivation of stimuli from the sense which has been lost, and thus a condition of mental instability is set up. This instability, however, is probably not so often the cause of the mental symptoms as the sense of helplessness and loss of touch with his surroundings, which tends to make those who are blind or deaf at first suspicious and finally examples of delusional insanity. The delusions in all of such cases are those of suspicion, the blind man imagining his wife is flirting with a rival in his very presence, the deaf man that his neighbours are laughing and talking about him and so on. Physical symptoms are rarely, if ever, associated with these cases, the condition being purely a psychical one.

Treatment.—The treatment of such a case depends more on the tactful sympathetic manner of the medical adviser than on diet or drugs. By gaining the confidence of your patient his suspicions become less and less acute and may in time wholly disappear. Want of tact, want of sympathy, and deceit on the part of those around him, however, will promptly cause the reappearance of all the old suspicions, so that in every such case we must explain things carefully to all those around our patient and ask their co-operation in restoring him to his right mind.

Prognosis.—Rapid recovery is to be expected in most cases but, as can be gathered from what has already been said, relapses are frequent in the majority of cases unless the utmost tact and care be exercised by the friends and relatives of the patient.

CHAPTER XI.

INSANITIES OF TOXIC ORIGIN.

Group I.—Insanities the Result of Toxines of Metabolic Origin.

The term "Metabolic Toxæmia" is, as Dr. Bruce admits, a vague and unscientific one for the reason that not only the nature of the toxines but the very toxines themselves are unknown. Probably the most important are the preurea bodies and perhaps the ethereal sulphates, as well as certain anæmic conditions where there is an accumulation of waste products in the body.

In all acute insanities, as I have all along endeavoured to impress on my readers, there is distinct evidence of metabolic disorder, but, in one type of disease, namely Acute Melancholia, metabolic toxæmia is most markedly present, and to such an extent that there can be but little doubt that the mental derangement is mainly, if not wholly, due to this deranged metabolism.

ACUTE MELANCHOLIA.

Definition. Acute Melancholia may be defined as a distinct physical disease, with definite physical symptoms, affecting mainly those in the decline of life and only rarely seen in adolescence when it is evidence of bad heredity. It is liable to recur and eventually end in a chronic delusional state.

Ætiology.—The chief predisposing cause is undoubtedly a bad heredity, but any weakening, fatiguing mental or physical conditions, such as overwork, anxiety, worry and deprivation of sleep may cause such a disorder. These latter conditions, leading, as they do, to derangements of metabolism which directly cause the mental condition, may be also cited as exciting causes.

Symptoms—Prodromata.—The onset of the disease is slow and insidious, and indefinite symptoms of ill-health, gastric disturbances, loss of weight and sleeplessness, are often present for months before any signs of mental symptoms are noticed. This prodromal period is one to which I would especially direct my reader's attention, for if it be recognised and the patient at once put under proper treatment, the chances are very great indeed that the attack may be stayed and the family perhaps saved from being tainted with the curse of insanity and all the horror and suffering which it entails.

Physical symptoms.—By the time mental symptoms manifest themselves all such cases are thin and poorly nourished owing to the lengthy prodromal period through which they have come. In the *acute stage of onset*, the tongue is furred and foul, appetite is usually deficient or wanting altogether, owing to loss of the digestive power of the gastric juices, but excessive thirst is almost invariably present. The pulse rate is rapid, irregular in force and rhythm, and the arterial tension, as a rule, is markedly increased. In pure uncomplicated cases there is no marked change in the leucocytes, both the total number per c.mm. and the percentages of the various types remaining about the normal; there is, however, always more or less anæmia present, due more to a deficiency in the amount of hæmoglobin than to a diminution in number of the red blood corpuscles.

The skin is hot and dry and the temperature is often slightly raised in the evenings. The urine is scanty and passed at long intervals, the urea excreted is generally markedly deficient in quantity and albumen is often present in small amounts. This falling-off in the amount of urine excreted is remarkable when one considers the amount of fluids such persons drink in the course of a single day, and is probably due to the water being broken up in the system, as in the *post mortem* on such cases the tissues are invariably abnormally dry. Restlessness and depression are marked at the onset of all such cases.

As the acute stage passes off, the restlessness and depression gradually disappear, the tongue cleans from the tip and edges, appetite gradually returns, there is less tendency to constipation and the gastric juice is more freely secreted and has greater digestive power. There are at no stage of the disease any signs of hyperleucocytosis and nothing abnormal is to be found in the corpuscles in uncomplicated cases. The pulse gradually becomes slower and more regular, and the arterial tension falls, while the skin becomes moister and gradually regains its elasticity. Occasionally one meets with profuse perspirations in such cases, somewhat resembling the crisis of acute specific diseases, but these are not very frequent and are generally accompanied by excessive urinary excretion and marked increase in the excretion of urea, which, in some cases, may rise to even 800 grains in the 24 hours.

Nervous System.—Sensibility to heat, touch and pain are very commonly diminished, more probably owing to the concentration of the whole faculty of attention on the feeling of extreme mental depression than to any failure in the peripheral enervation, and the special senses of taste and smell are frequently disordered. The organic reflexes remain as a rule under control, the diminution in micturition being directly due to diminished excretion, but the superficial and deep reflexes are frequently found to be increased. Voluntary muscular movements are sluggish and the powers of fine co-ordination are impaired. As the acute stage passes off, voluntary movement becomes easier and more natural, sensibility is gradually restored and by degrees the patient returns to his normal condition.

Mental Symptoms.—The mental condition in cases of acute melancholia varies greatly in intensity. In an average case there is invariably well-marked depression which the presence of marked hallucinations may increase greatly in amount. There is as a rule a varying degree of confusion with a loss of the power of cognition, due probably, in great measure, to the deranged attention which is wholly occupied in considering the wretched state in which the patient fancies he is situated. Vivid hallucinations of hearing are often present and may give rise to delusions, but, as a rule, in the acute stage these are masked to a certain extent by the confusion and only become pronounced at the later stages of the disease.

In every case all sense of personal cleanliness and order is lost, there being apparently no thought or care for anything but the condition of mental depression which occupies the whole mind of the patient.

Loss of self-control is an invariable concomitant and is evidenced by extreme restlessness and impulsive movements, which are commonly due to fright caused by terrifying hallucinations.

The attention, as already noted, is wholly subjective, and self-control and memory on this account cannot be tested, and speech, when present, is jerky and spasmodic, though occasionally mutism is met with. Insomnia is invariably present in all cases.

The acute stage may last from 2—3 weeks to 2—3 months and occasionally ends in a rapid recovery with critical discharges as already noted, though, as a rule, it gradually merges into a sub-acute condition, the physical and mental symptoms gradually fading in intensity. This sub-acute stage may gradually improve and end in recovery, but relapses are frequent, all the symptoms of the acute stages then returning, and at times the condition passes into one of chronic depression with symptoms of nutritive failure.

When recovery occurs, memory of what has happened during the acute stage is, as a rule, but vague, and often absent altogether, though memory of the previous life is unimpaired. The physical condition invariably improves before the mental, the whole course of the disease and appearance of the patient reminding one of an exhausting physical disease.

When a state of chronic depression ensues, the patient remains thin and unhealthy looking. Digestion remains weak and the patient suffers from dyspepsia, anorexia and constipation. The pulse is weak and thready and the extremities are cyanosed and cold. Trophic changes are evidenced by the dry pigmented skin, the brittle lustreless hair and nails and the great tendency there is for such patients to be carried off by pulmonary tuberculosis. The excretion of urine and urea is markedly irregular, and there is general impairment of sensibility and lack of normal tone throughout the body.

Death may occur in the acute stage, the patient passing into a typhoid state, or suicide may occur in any of the three stages, though most commonly during the acute stage of onset owing to the sudden impulses so frequently met with in that stage.

Diagnosis.—This depends largely upon the clinical symptoms, thus physically we have the disordered alimentary tract, the rapid irregular pulse, the high arterial tension, the deficient excretion of urea and urine and the absence of hyperleucocytosis, while mentally we have the extreme mental depression with, as a rule, only a comparatively small amount of confusion.

Treatment.—In the stage of acute onset rest in bed and careful nursing by night and day are essential, while the condition of the digestive organs indicates an absolutely simple diet. Milk is the best food in all such conditions and should be given in small quantities and at frequent intervals. Water should be given freely and the patient allowed as much as he can drink, with a view to assist in the excretion of waste products from the system as well as to meet the apparent destruction of water in the body. Constipation should be alleviated by large saline enemata.

As the condition improves, additions may be made to the dietary with caution, purin-free foods such as bread, butter, sugar, eggs, rice and potatoes being added gradually at first, and later very weak tea, white meat and fish.

Drugs.—For insomnia in this condition paraldehyde is undoubtedly the best drug we have. It should not be given every night but ʒii be given one night and then two nights allowed to elapse and the drug again given on the third night if necessary. In this way the risk of establishing a "drug habit" is avoided, and nature is given an opportunity to restore the natural powers of sleep. Sulphonal should never be given in acute melancholia as it interferes with the elaboration of urea from the nitrogenous waste products of the body. When the acute stage is over, tonics such as quinine, strychnine and dilute acids, should be exhibited and the patient made to take exercise, which should, however, be begun by degrees and be carefully regulated so as to avoid fatiguing the patient.

Prognosis.—In adult life the prognosis is as a rule good, most cases recovering within six months, but in cases occurring in late adult life or in old age the prognosis is less favourable, the sub-acute stage being apt to be prolonged and at times pass into a condition of chronic depression with delusions. In adolescence the immediate prognosis is good, but the condition is very liable to recur and such recurrent attacks of melancholia are often the precursors of chronic delusional insanity.

INSANITY OF MYXŒDEMA.

In all persons suffering from myxœdema there is some mental change, in some perhaps so slight that it may be passed over unnoticed, while in others it may be so marked as to call for special treatment. One must, however, always remember there is a mental as well as a physical side to this condition, and not allow the prominence of the physical symptoms to make us forget the mental aspect of the case, as in this way some unforeseen accident may occur which a little care might otherwise have avoided.

Ætiology.—The condition is in all cases due to the failure of the performance of the normal functions of the thyroid gland. It usually appears about the age of thirty to thirty-five and more commonly affects women.

Physical Symptoms.—Only a brief résumé of these will be given here and for further details any medical text-book may be consulted. The hands become broad and "spadelike" and the power of finely co-ordinated movement is lost. The hair and nails become brittle, the former often coming out in handfuls and leaving the patient bald, whilst the latter are always splitting and breaking. The teeth are very prone to decay and trophic changes are common throughout the body. The fatty tissues under the skin are involved, the skin of the face becomes swollen and waxy, the swelling being elastic and unaffected by pressure or gravity. Irregular thickenings of the subdermal tissues occur in various regions, especially the axillary and the supra-clavicular, while the abdomen becomes large and pendulous from the same cause. The mucous membranes become involved also and the tongue is large and thickened. The pulse is, as a rule, very slow and such cases are constantly complaining of chilliness and are very susceptible to alterations of temperature. Anæmia is well marked in advanced cases and women invariably suffer from amenorrhœa. Constipation is almost invariably present, and hæmorrhages from mucous membranes are by no means uncommon.

Mental Symptoms.—The early stages of myxœdema are invariably marked by a steadily progressive mental deterioration. Movement and thought become slower and there is failure of general comprehension. Memory becomes defective for recent events, the power for work is diminished, mistakes are frequent and outbursts of irritability are common. These patients, as a rule, are fully aware of this failure in their mental powers and frequently complain about it, while with many it produces a condition of marked depression.

If left untreated the general lethargy increases and the patient suffers from overwhelming drowsiness. He loses all interest in his personal appearance and day by day he becomes more sluggish and clumsy in his movements and more and more easily fatigued. He loses all interest in his surroundings and pays no heed to the wants of others. The greater majority of such cases suffer from a species of mild depression with vague ill-defined fears for which they cannot account, though, in some cases, the early irritability developes into acute excitement. In advanced cases marked delusions and hallucinations are present, but such cases are rarely suicidal or homicidal.

Diagnosis.—The diagnosis is a matter of comparative ease, though, when acute mental symptoms have developed, the general condition may possibly be overlooked. Bright's disease is most apt to be confounded with it, but close examination reveals many points of distinction.

Pathology.—In all cases the thyroid gland is either atrophied or diseased. In the earlier stages there is a small celled infiltration into the walls of the vesicles and the gland gradually passes into a condition of fibrous atrophy, small groups of cells and colloid masses being scattered throughout the fibrous tissue.

Treatment.—It is wise to begin with small doses of thyroid, and gradually increase the amount if necessary, firstly, because small doses may be sufficient for recovery, and secondly, because with larger doses untoward results are likely to occur, 3—5 minims of liquor thyroidei (B. P.) or 3 grains of thyroideum siccum daily are quite sufficient for a commencement. During this treatment the patient should be kept in bed, and the temperature recorded daily in the morning and evening, the pulse rate being also taken. If in a few days no improvement is seen, the dose must be gradually increased, but in no case should the drug be pressed with the idea of hastening recovery, as such a proceeding is most risky. Persistent frontal headache, dizziness, increased excitement, rapid heart's action, diarrhœa, fever, urticaria, etc., etc., are indications for reducing the dose. If all goes well, the physical and mental conditions improve rapidly, many undergoing complete recovery in about three months, but such patients must be made to understand that it will be necessary to continue taking thyroid throughout their lives, though usually comparatively small doses suffice ; the amount necessary for each patient, however, is only ascertainable by careful observation.

Prognosis.—If left untreated, such cases go from bad to worse, death ultimately resulting from coma or some intercurrent disease. If treatment has been begun early in the course of the disease, complete recovery may occur, but in the majority of these cases such is not the case, and there remains a certain amount of physical and mental enfeeblement, rendering them unfit to perform arduous duties.

DELUSIONAL INSANITY.

Under this head I am grouping conditions variously described by other authors as progressive systematised insanity ; mania of persecution ; monomanias of pride and grandeur ; megalomania and paranoia. This last condition is described by many as one of the forms of "Dementia Præcox," katatonia and hebephrenia being the other two. A little consideration, however, convinces one of the error of this, for paranoia is of total different origin from either katatonia or hebephrenia, which are both due to bacterial toxæmias, and moreover except that they all tend to affect largely young adults of marked neurotic heredity they have not a single feature in common.

Dementia Præcox too is a misleading term to apply to any of these conditions, for though most of the cases occur in early adult life, their incidence is not wholly confined to this period, cases by no means infrequently being postponed to much later age periods. For these reasons therefore, and because the conditions mentioned above as described by various authors seem to me to belong to very much the same physical and mental states, I am ignoring the term Dementia Præcox and grouping these various conditions under the one head of "Delusional Insanity."*

Many forms of insanity tend to become complicated with delusions if the patient does not recover, but such delusions are mere indications of the chronicity of the disease and of the mental impairment, and their character is wholly different, as they are more changeable and fleeting, the patient has not arguments to bring forward in support of them, and they do not influence the whole habits and life of the patient, as is the case in the condition which I am now about to describe. In such cases too we have the history of the case, and in many instances physical symptoms also, which enable us to distinguish what condition we are dealing with.

Definition.—These conditions may be defined typically as mental states of marked delusions, generally of systematised persecution, at times combined with grandiose delusions, such delusions affecting the whole life of the patient and being supported by fierce argument if their truth be in any way questioned.

---

* I see in the Medico-Psychological Journal for January 1912, that this view is now commonly held among alienists in Great Britain. Among them Dementia Præcox, pure and simple, is always understood to imply katatonia, and is never used, unqualified, when referring to either paranoia or hebephrenia.

Ætiology.—As already noted hereditary taint is by far the most common predisposing cause, a history of this being obtainable in well over 50% of cases affected, a badly regulated education, unhygienic surroundings, want of proper care and supervision when children, sexual and alcoholic excesses and venereal disease all tend to predispose towards an attack though practically nothing is known as to the exciting causes.

The disease affects the sexes equally and its incidence is most marked in adolescence.

Symptoms.—It is essentially a disease of failure of nutrition, with vague symptoms of malaise and sensory disturbances which gradually develope into hallucinations and delusions which are invariably of a persecutory type.

In many instances the disease begins gradually and passes unnoticed until attention is drawn to it by an assault, or some other crime, committed by the patient as the result of his delusions. In other cases, however, there may be an acute attack, with symptoms similar to those of acute metabolic poisoning, which may either pass into a chronic delusional condition or from which there may be apparent recovery, the chronic delusional state coming on gradually and months may pass before it is sufficiently developed to attract attention.

Physical Symptoms.—(*a*) *The acute onset* as a rule resembles an attack of acute melancholia except for the presence of marked delusions. There is dyspepsia and anorexia. The pulse is fast and of high tension and the temperature is frequently above normal. The urinary excretion is diminished and frequently contains traces of albumen, while the excretion of chlorides and urea is markedly diminished. The leucocytosis is never raised nor are there ever any changes in the percentages of the various leucocytic elements. (*b*) *With the stage of chronic delusions* there are well marked physical symptoms. The patient is thin and sallow and has a furtive, suspicious expression. There is invariably more or less dyspepsia with furred tongue, foul breath and discomfort after meals. The heart's action is slow and feeble, but readily accelerated, and there is a tendency to syncope, while the arterial tension is slightly increased. Leucocytosis is almost invariably below the average. The excretion of urine is increased and with it there is an increase in the chlorides and urea excreted. The temperature is irregular showing occasional unexplainable rises which may be accompanied by indefinite complaints of malaise and discomfort. Sensory disturbances are frequent and as a rule the patient looks on them as modes of persecution employed by his enemies to annoy or injure him. The pupils may be unequal but react to light and accommodation.

Mental Symptoms.—(*a*) *Acute onset.* Depression with a certain amount of confusion is invariably present, and in nearly all cases there are marked hallucinations of hearing and frequently delusions of persecution. Self-control is diminished, the patient, as a rule, being frightened and subject to sudden impulses. The memory, both for past and present events, is impaired and attention to surroundings is in abeyance, owing to its being bound up in the feelings and sufferings of the patient, *i.e.*, subject-consciousness is greatly increased at the expense of object-consciousness. Insomnia is invariably present.

Such cases may at times undergo apparent recovery, while in others there may be frequent attacks of this description before the onset of the delusional state, in which case there are marked hallucinations present and persisting between the attacks. Other cases again seem to pass directly from the acute attack into the chronic delusional state, though as a rule some considerable time elapses before this condition becomes apparent.

(*b*) *The condition of chronic delusions* begins as a rule with hallucinations of hearing which may at first be recognised as such by the patient though in time they gain complete sway over him and the other special senses become involved too. As judgment fails these hallucinations give rise to delusions, in support of which the patient has elaborate arguments always ready and which govern his whole life and conduct. The patient's mood is very variable in this stage being at various times depressed, irritable, sulky or truculent in one and the same case. Cognition is never affected nor is confusion ever noticed in such cases, but hallucinations are invariably present. These hallucinations at first are mainly those of hearing, the patient imagining people or "voices" are abusing him, or making accusations against him, or repeating his thoughts aloud, etc., etc. Disorders of taste and smell give rise to delusions, anent poison and foul gases being blown into the room, while derangements of sensation similarly cause delusions of hypnotism, electricity, etc.,

etc. As a rule these imaginary persecutions are all ascribed to the machinations of some one person or sect, and in time every one with whom the patient comes in contact is supposed to be influenced by his enemy. Along with these sensory hallucinations and delusions of persecution one sees in almost every case delusions of a grandiose type, due probably to failure of judgment and a deficient object-consciousness. As a result of these delusions all sorts of impracticable schemes are promulgated, one patient has discovered the elixir of life, another is going to convert all Brahmins to Mohammedanism, a third has found a means of converting stones and rubbish into gold, etc., etc. In every case the patient is full of hope and convinced of the success of his plans, and when they miscarry cites it as but another example of the persecution he endures. In cases where there is much depression the delusions are at times of a melancholic type and often religious in nature, and in such cases we must always be ready to prevent attempts at suicide. Self-control is never markedly impaired in these conditions and patients generally can control their own actions. Assaults, however, are common and are due to the delusions, the patient being cognisant of his actions and laying his plans carefully beforehand as a rule, though at times the action may have been unpremeditated and then usually is due to an auditory hallucination, the reason being in both cases either a desire for revenge on his enemies or to rid himself from their constant persecution. The faculty of attention is good and the patients converse sensibly on any subject apart from their delusions, memory also remains unimpaired. Insomnia is a common complaint in these cases and is due as a rule to the sensory disturbances which are more marked commonly at night.

Diagnosis.—In such cases the main points which help us in our diagnosis are the history of the case and the fixity and character of the delusions, as well as the comparatively normal mentalisation of the patient except on the subject of these delusions.

Treatment.—In the acute stage rest in bed and a fluid diet is indicated, but in the later stages nothing can be done beyond giving attention to the bodily health and exerting careful supervision over the patient to prevent his committing assaults on other persons.

Prognosis.—Recovery from the mental condition is hopeless in such cases and can never be looked for. There is, however, no risk to life and as a rule but little mental deterioration, except in a certain number of adolescent cases of marked neurotic heredity who rapidly become demented.

CHRONIC METABOLIC TOXÆMIA.

In the chapter dealing with the non-toxic insanities I have dealt with the mental symptoms arising from conditions of brain anæmia due to occlusion of the cerebral arteries and I there mentioned that the conditions which caused this condition of the arteries were quite capable of producing mental symptoms from their action on the cortical centres. It is this last condition with which I propose to deal now.

Ætiology.—This condition practically never occurs before middle life, as a rule commencing about the climacteric. In a large percentage of such patients a history of a previous mental attack is obtainable, and almost invariably this attack has been one of depression. A history of excessive alcoholism or drug taking is obtainable in a large number of cases and may be either a symptom, the drug having been taken to alleviate gastric discomfort, or a cause, the continued use of the drug producing metabolic disorder by deranging the functions of the intestines, liver and kidneys.

Symptoms.—Physical Symptoms.—The condition being wholly due to the accumulation of waste products in the system it is but little to be wondered at that the symptoms both physical and mental approximate closely to those of chronic melancholia. The onset is gradual and characterised by dyspepsia, anorexia and constipation. The patient's appearance alters, the skin assuming a dull pallor owing to anæmia and œdema of the subcutaneous tissues. The pulse is thready and of very high tension, and there is deficiency both in the number of the red blood corpuscles and in the percentage of hæmoglobin, though there is no alteration in the leucocytosis. Attacks of palpitation are frequently seen early in the disease and as a rule are accompanied by vertigo and severe headaches. Sensory disturbances too are frequent, the patient complaining of fornication, etc., which often give rise to delusions of persecution.

Mental Symptoms.—The mental state belonging to this condition is invariably one of depression combined with hallucinations and delusions. Confusion is a fairly prominent symptom in most cases, and judgment and memory are impaired. Attention too is deranged and what little remains is so largely self-centred that it is impossible to attract the patient's attention for long, and conversation as a result is difficult. Attempts at suicide have to be guarded against in this condition.

Diagnosis.—The age and history of the patient and the physical and mental symptoms form an entity which in typical cases there is but little difficulty in diagnosing.

Treatment.—Rest, light nourishing diet with plenty of fluid ingesta and gentle regulated exercise are indicated in these conditions.

Prognosis.—In all such cases the prognosis is very bad. The patients are liable to be suddenly carried off by some intercurrent disease, and in those cases who do live some degree of mental deterioration invariably remains and, as a rule, the last years of their lives drag on in a state of more or less marked secondary dementia.

CHAPTER XII.

INSANITIES OF TOXIC ORIGIN.—(*Contd.*)

Group II.—Insanities in which there is evidence of Bacterial Toxæmia.

INSANITIES due to bacterial toxæmias are much more serious conditions than those due to purely exhaustive or metabolic causes. An invariable concomitant of such conditions is a hyperleucocytosis with a high polymorphonuclear percentage in the early stages, and whenever such a condition is found to prevail one can be sure one is dealing with a case of bacterial toxæmia. As a rule the most characteristic symptom of the group is excitement, associated with mental confusion, depression or elevation, while relapses are frequently met with in these conditions. In practically all cases after an attack of this sort evidences of toxæmia persist in the blood for years after even apparent complete recovery has taken place, and this, combined with the frequency with which relapses occur, can but lead one to the conclusion that perfect recovery from such conditions very rarely occurs.

EXCITED MELANCHOLIA.

Until very recent years this condition has always been regarded as a type or variety of melancholia, and indeed this view is still held by many of the older members of the medical profession. There is undoubtedly a superficial resemblance between it and what I have described as acute melancholia, but an examination of the physical symptoms, and an examination more especially of the blood can lead to but one conclusion and that is that excited melancholia and acute melancholia are as separate and distinct diseases as are typhus and enteric fever, and that they should be similarly diagnosed and treated as two separate and distinct diseases.

Ætiology.—This condition is most liable to occur in late adult life and is seen frequently during the climacteric period in women. As a rule heredity and alcoholic excesses have but little connection with this condition, long-continued worry, excessive mental strain, and the natural failure of the vital powers as life declines being the chief predisposing factors, while in all cases the exciting cause is a toxæmia of bacterial origin. How or whence the toxæmia arises is at present undetermined, but the probability is that the seat of infection is the intestine, and that the infection itself is caused by some of the saprophitic bacteria of the body becoming virulent and secreting toxines which act directly on the nervous tissues.

Symptoms—Prodromata.—In practically every case a history of great physical and mental strain is obtainable. As a result of this the patient becomes dyspeptic, sleepless and anæmic, and complains of physical and mental lassitude, for which he frequently seeks medical aid. This condition gradually goes from bad to worse, the patient becomes unable to carry out his ordinary duties and unable to rest, and, if medical advice has not been previously sought, he is now driven to call for our aid.

Physical Symptoms.—The patient is always thin and badly nourished and his expression is invariably one of misery or anxiety, and often of fear. Flatulent dyspepsia with disinclination for food and drink, sometimes so marked as to necessitate artificial feeding, are very common, and constipation is invariably a marked feature of such cases. The temperature is as a rule irregularly febrile, the elevations usually occurring in the evening. The pulse is fast and weak and the arterial tension is low. Anæmia is invariably present and is accompanied by a hyperleucocytosis with a marked increase in the polymorphonuclear percentage. Trophic changes are evidenced by papular rashes, which the patient picks causing unsightly sores, or by erysipelatous attacks which at times seem to take the place of exacerbations of the mental symptoms. The urinary excretion remains fairly normal both in quality and quantity. Sensibility is frequently impaired, formications or flushings of heat and cold being often complained of, while sensibility, both to temperature and pain, seems diminished. The organic, superficial and deep reflexes are as a rule all unaffected, though irritability of the motor area of the cortex is shown in restlessness, slight loss of co-ordination and fine tremors in the muscles of the face and hands.

Mental Symptoms.—The main mental symptoms are acute depression and anxiety, with practically no confusion or loss of consciousness ; as a rule confusion is but rarely seen and when present it is transient and coincident with the acme of the acute attack. Hallucinations and delusions are but seldom present, never in typical cases, and when they do occur are transitory and of little moment. Subject-consciousness is markedly increased while object-consciousness is diminished, though not so markedly that attention cannot be obtained but there is no capacity for occupation of any sort. Self-control is markedly diminished as shown by the constant restlessness, noisy declamation and attempts at suicide. The powers of speech and of comprehending written and spoken language remain as a rule unimpaired. Insomnia is invariably present during the attack and often persists after apparent recovery.

Diagnosis.—Acute Melancholia is the chief condition likely to trouble us here. Dr. Bruce has tabulated the distinctive features of these two conditions most clearly and I quote his table here for the benefit of my readers.

	Acute Melancholia.	Excited Melancholia.
Physical.		
(*a*) Alimentary.	Marked disturbance	Less disturbance.
(*b*) Hæmopoietic	Moderate leucocytosis.	Hyperleucocytosis.
(*c*) Urinary.	Excretion of urine and urea deficient.	No abnormality detected.
Mental.	Mental confusion with vivid hallucinations which affect the conduct.	Little or no mental confusion. Hallucinations not necessarily present.

In acute melancholia too the patients as a rule are listless and quiet, whereas in excited melancholia the patient lives in a condition of constant restlessness, wandering aimlessly about, twisting or rubbing the hands, picking at the skin, hair or clothes, and ejaculating or groaning in a rhythmical somewhat staccato manner.

Treatment.—In the acute stage complete rest in bed and a light diet are essential.

Calomel and a saline purge should be administered as soon as possible in such cases, and, if necessary, repeated in 4 or 5 days time. Hydrarg. subchlor. grs. iii followed by mag. sulph. ʒiv or a seidlitz powder after four hours is what I usually order. On the subsidence of the acute symptoms general tonics with mild regulated exercise, and a full and plentiful dietary are indicated, and we should always endeavour to keep the patient's attention off himself by mild amusements or occupations, though avoiding anything likely to cause fatigue. In some cases small doses of nepenthe given 3 or 4 times daily have very beneficial results, but if improvement does not occur in a day or two it is wiser to stop the drug as otherwise an opium habit may be started. In the more acute cases sulphonal grs. x combined with potassium bromide grs. xxx and administered twice or thrice daily has often most excellent sedative results, though both these drugs tend to increase gastric disorder and still further lower the nutrition.

Prognosis.—The prognosis is in all cases a bad one, many cases continuing in a state of chronic depression for years. Recovery is seldom complete but partial recoveries are not uncommon, though such cases are invariably subject to constant relapses.

MANIACAL EXCITEMENT WITH CONFUSION (ACUTE MANIA).

Mania, strictly speaking, is applicable to but one outstanding symptom and that is excitement, but in practice it is also used to designate a distinct mental condition which many authors subdivide into various forms. As pointed out by Dr. Bruce, however, a careful consideration of the physical symptoms present in this condition of acute toxæmia associated with maniacal excitement, can lead to but one conclusion, namely, that the disease is one and the same whether it lasts for a fortnight or a lifetime, whether it is recurrent or non-recurrent, and whether the symptoms are so severe as to deserve the term delirious or so mild as to be called sub-acute.

As with all toxic conditions, so in this disease we have the symptoms modified by various factors such as the individual power of resistance to the toxines, the virulence of the bacteria, and these factors themselves are affected by climatic and various other conditions. Thus the various conditions described by so many authors have arisen, owing partly to their classifying disease on a symptomatological instead of an ætiological basis and partly to their having given undue prominence to mental at the expense of physical symptoms.

Dr. Bruce divides "Mania" into two classes, *viz.* :—

(*a*). " A condition of mental excitement, associated during its early stages with complete loss of consciousness (*i.e.*, confusion), with hallucinations and illusions, with complete loss of the powers of attention and memory, with incoherence of speech and loss of comprehension of language spoken or written; while on the physical side, there are evidences of very acute toxæmia." This condition he describes under the term " Acute Mania or Excitement with Confusion."

(*b*). " A condition of excitement without confusion but rather associated with a hyperacute consciousness without hallucinations or delusions. The powers of attention are not lost, but wander loosely from subject to subject. The memory is often very acute. The speech, though rambling, disjointed and inconsequent, is not, in itself, incoherent. The patient readily understands spoken or written language, and although the writing may be fantastic in style and in composition, the power of writing is not lost. Physically the symptoms of toxæmia are much less severe." This type is described by Dr. Bruce as " Folie Circulaire or Excitement without Confusion."

In some cases of Acute Mania, when the condition has lasted for a considerable period, there is a return of consciousness with some capacity for attention and observation, and as a result the condition, viewed from the mental aspect, is not markedly dissimilar from Folie Circulaire and mistakes in diagnosis are liable to occur. Notwithstanding this the distinction between the two diseases seems to me so clearly established that I propose adhering to Dr. Bruce's classification.

and describing conditions of maniacal excitement under these two heads alone.

Typhoid or delirious mania is undoubtedly a misnomer as any toxic insanity, whether metabolic or toxæmic, may terminate in such a state and as a rule there is a rapidly fatal termination to such cases. Simple mania too is a misleading term being equally applicable to the early stages of Acute Mania or Folie Circulaire.

Acute Mania.—Such conditions are most typical when affecting adults, and, as a rule, cases affecting adults are more continuous and less liable to remissions and exacerbations which are so common at other age periods.

Ætiology.—Hereditary predisposition is a well marked factor in the production of this condition, British statistics showing a history of neurotic taint in at least 50% of the cases and the presumption is that a similar condition prevails in India. The exciting cause in practically all cases is some condition which has lowered the natural resistive powers of the patient, such as mental worry or shock, bodily privation, unhealthy surroundings, alcoholic excesses and, in women, childbirth.

Symptoms—Prodromata.—The onset usually is gradual, the patient complaining of malaise, insomnia, restlessness, and inability to concentrate his attention and thoughts for any length of time. Perversions of affection are common, patients taking unaccountable dislikes to relatives and friends. Headaches are constant in practically every case, and flatulent dyspepsia is a constant cause of complaint.

In a few instances the acute attack is suppressed, the patient passing from the prodromal stage to an irritable moody condition with a certain amount of confusion, and later on the developement of delusions.

As a rule, however, an acute attack succeeds the above prodromal symptoms and may be either acute in its onset or supervene gradually.

Physical Symptoms.—The patient's face is drawn and pale, the eyes are bright and staring and the pupils dilated but reacting to both light and accommodation. The temperature varies according to the stage of the disease, in the stage of acute onset and during exacerbations and recurrences the temperature is irregularly febrile, but after a week or so it becomes subnormal and remains thus throughout the attack and even after apparent recovery it may still be found about a degree below the normal. Paradoxical temperatures (*i.e.*, temperatures with their maxima occurring in the morning) are common in but by no means characteristic of this condition.

Gastric derangement is profound in the early stages of this condition, the teeth and lips are covered with sordes, the tongue is furred and foul, and for the first few weeks there is marked distaste for food, though, as a rule, excessive thirst is present. After this time, however, even though much of the excitement still remains, the appetite returns and with it the digestive powers, the patient eating ravenously and digesting practically everything. These altered states of appetite are explained by Dr. Bruce, who has found that at the onset of the attack the secretion of the gastric juices is practically abolished while at a later stage the gastric secretions are plentiful and very active.

The heart is as a rule normal, the pulse at the onset may be increased in rate and slightly irregular, but it is never so fast as in a case of excited melancholia and rarely exceeds 100 beats per minute. If the attack is of long duration cardiac weakness may be seen and a tendency to syncope arise. The skin generally is dry, but excessive perspiration may affect the palms of the hands and the soles of the feet. Trophic changes are manifested by various rashes and pustular eruptions, while the hair and nails become dry and brittle, the hair at times standing on end and adding a finishing touch to the physical representation so typical of the mental condition.

Urinary excretion is scanty at the beginning of the attack, but the nitrogenous excretion is increased, probably owing to the incessant muscular movements, later in the disease however the urinary excretion is generally well above the normal. The excretion of the chlorides in the urine is diminished in the acute stage, but, as improvement sets in, there is, as a rule, a sudden rise in the amount excreted, the rise being in proportion to the amount of chlorides ingested during the acute stage of the disease.

Sensibility to heat and pain are diminished, but the sense of touch is as a rule hyperacute, as are also all the special senses except that of taste which is often deficient. Superficial reflexes are generally slightly increased but the tendon reflexes as a rule are unaffected and the organic reflexes remain under control unless the attack be very severe. There is never paralysis or weakness of the voluntary muscles, and the inco-ordination which is seen in all cases and especially affects the facial muscles, is due to irritation of the cortical centres.

The blood presents characteristic features in this condition and I shall quote here from Dr. Bruce's results, for, though I have examined a small number of cases myself, my results are too few to generalise upon and they accord closely to those cited by Dr. Bruce.

In the early part of the acute stages there is invariably a hyperleucocytosis amounting to 18,000 or 20,000 per c. m. m. and the polymorphonuclear percentage is never below 70 per cent. After a few days this hyperleucocytosis falls, occasionally to 10,000 per c. m. m. but never lower, and as a rule to 14,000 or 15,000 per c. m. m., and this fall is accompanied by a fall in the polymorphonuclears to 60 per cent. or even lower whilst a corresponding rise occurs in the lymphocytes and a smaller rise in the percentage of the eosinophiles, though this last is not an invariable condition. Whenever distinct mental improvement sets in the leucocytosis again rises and with it the polymorphonuclear percentage which is practically always above 70 per cent. As recovery becomes complete the polymorphonuclear percentage again falls to between 60 and 70 per cent., but the hyperleucocytosis persists for long, probably indefinitely, and the presumption is that it is a protective leucocytosis necessary to maintain an efficient immunity against the source of the disease which is still in the body of the patient.

When recovery does not occur, the leucocytosis as a rule falls, and with it the polymorphonuclear percentage may fall to as low as even 30 or 40 per cent.

As a rule recovery occurs within six months of the onset of the symptoms, the severity of the attack gradually passing off, sleep returning and the patient increasing in weight. Occasionally there is an unhealthy puffy appearance about the patient, somewhat similar to that seen in patients who have recovered from some septicæmia. At times, however, the patient passes into a condition of chronic excitement, with physical symptoms akin to that of the acute state but less in severity. In a very small number of cases the acute condition passes into a state of delirious or typhoid mania, which is characterised by delirious excitement followed by a stage of exhaustion in which the patient lies helplessly picking the bed clothes, with dry, cracked lips and tongue, and sordes on the teeth. The patient wastes rapidly in this condition, the urine and fæces are passed unconsciously and diarrhœa is a great source of trouble. Hypostatic congestion of the lungs occurs and death is simply then a question of a few days.

Mental Symptoms.—Loss of self-control, mental excitement and marked confusion are characteristic of this condition, and are, as a rule, associated with loss of the power of cognition both of place and person, loss of the faculty of attention, incoherent speech, insomnia and extreme motor restlessness. Such patients too are as a rule very emotional, readily changing from laughter to tears or anger, but usually a condition of well being and excitement prevails, tears being gusty and merely superficial and not due to any lasting condition. Hallucinations both of sight and hearing occur in most cases and may be associated with delusions.

In cases where gradual recovery occurs, the symptoms lose their severity by degrees and gradually short periods of comparative sanity occur, as a rule being seen in the morning after a good night's rest. These periods gradually become more and more prolonged until, with occasional moments of loss of self-control, the greater part of the day is passed in quiet and sanity.

Where the acute stage passes into a state of chronic restlessness, consciousness returns and the patient is fully aware of all that passes, but there is no return of self-control or of ability for work of any sort, and in many such cases destructive tendencies are marked, clothes and furniture being destroyed, while the patients are readily pleased or irritated, and liable to impulses of an aggressive or erotic type. Such cases may drag on for years in this state, until a mild dementia arrests the worst symptoms and renders the patients fit for ordinary unskilled labour under supervision.

In the comparatively rare state of "typhoid mania" delirious excitement is seen at the onset, but this gradually passes into a more or less comatose condition which continues till death occurs.

Relapses and recurrences are frequently seen in this form of insanity, definite periods of sanity occurring in the latter cases between the attacks. In the continuous attacks immunity seems to be more slowly established but, once it is established, the effects seem to be much more lasting than in the recurrent cases, where immunity is much more rapidly established but seems to be of only short duration. These differences in immunity periods are explained by Dr. Bruce as being due to variations in the resistive powers of the patients or to differences in the origin and virulence of the toxines causing the disease.

Diagnosis.—The only conditions likely to be mistaken for this are the elevated stage of "folie circulaire" and the excitement present in the onset of so many of the other insanities. In the former case the lack of confusion and the hyperacute state of the sensibilities serves to distinguish folie circulaire, but in the latter conditions it may be necessary to temporise for a time until the condition makes itself clear.

Treatment.—Rest in bed and careful nursing both by day and night are essential in the acute stages of the disease. Thorough evacuation of the bowels preferably by calomel and a saline purge should be obtained. The dietary should be light and as far as possible fluid, and, when necessary, artificially digested, and should be administered every two or three hours with a liberal allowance of stimulants. Large saline enemata are often most beneficial in such cases or, if these are not retained, subcutaneous injection of one to two pints produces equally good results. Insomnia is most troublesome in the acute stages and the continuous hot bath at 100° F. is often marvellous in its effects. The benefits derived from a hot bath, however, are evanescent and every third or fourth night hypnotics may be required to produce a sound night's sleep and I infinitely prefer paraldehyde in such cases given in large doses, even up to ʒiv if necessary. Hypnotics, however, should be used as little as possible for they tend to augment the gastric derangements and still further diminish the self-control, and by stupefying the patient render him dirty in his habits.

Prognosis.—As a rule in most cases the immediate prognosis is fairly good, though the frequency with which relapses and recurrences are seen must render us guarded in our ultimate prognosis, which is in truth far from hopeful. Rapid emaciation, the presence of auditory hallucinations and marked degeneracy, as evidenced by disregard of the calls of nature or the eating of filth, usually indicate an unfavourable prognosis. If the attack occurs early in life subsequent attacks are to be expected as a rule, especially if there be a markedly neurotic history or some definite cause for the illness. In delirious or typhoid mania the prognosis is most unfavourable, death occurring in nearly every case.

The various types of mania described by the older writers on psychiatry are similar to the above description but modified by variations in individual resistance or virulence in toxines as already mentioned.

The recurrent form is especially liable to occur in adolescents and is characterised by its comparatively sudden onset, its short duration and rapid convalescence, but it presents no other features beyond what are seen in the ordinary cases already described.

In cases of *mania following on the puerperium* there are always very marked symptoms of toxæmia present. In some cases, where the uterus is tender or the lochia fœtid or suppressed, there can be no doubt that the uterine cavity is the source of this infection, but in others this is not the case, and in these latter relapses are more frequent and there is the tendency to persistent hyperleucocytosis after recovery which is seen in other cases of acute mania. In mania following after the puerperal state both the physical and mental symptoms are very acute and the patient is apt to be subject to impulses, and infanticide and suicide have both to be carefully guarded against. The treatment is the same as in other cases of acute mania, with attention to the uterine condition superadded, *i.e.*, curetting and douching when necessary.

The prognosis, in cases due to a septic uterus, is as a rule much more favourable, recovery occurring in about 70 per cent., while relapses are much less common; where however the toxæmia is not palpably due to an infected uterine cavity one should be guarded, as the prognosis in these cases is much the same as for ordinary cases of acute mania.

Puerperal Insanity is a term better left unused. Any type of insanity may follow on the puerperal condition and none are peculiar to it. It is but small wonder that cases do occur as its sequelæ, when one considers the exhaustion and pain of parturition, the loss of blood and the liability to septic infection which occur in this condition. The last of these is, and can be, the only true exciting cause of the insanity, the others being more predisposing factors, owing to the exhaustion and diminution of the resistive powers caused by them.

CHAPTER XIII.

INSANITIES OF TOXIC ORIGIN.—(*Contd.*)

Group II.—Insanities in which there is evidence of Bacterial Toxœmia—(Contd.)

FOLIE CIRCULAIRE.

Definition.—Folie Circulaire may be defined as a mental condition characterised by alternating attacks of elevation and depression, though at times one or other stage of the disease may be suppressed or so transient as to escape notice. Confusion, hallucinations and delusions are conspicuous by their absence in this disease. The condition as a rule commences in adolescence or early adult life, rarely originating at other age periods.

Ætiology.—Heredity plays a marked part in the production of this condition, about 70 per cent. of such cases having a marked hereditary taint. There is, in most cases, no appearance of physical derangement to be made out, and, as a rule, neither moral nor physical causes seem to play an important part as ætiological factors.

For purposes of description this condition is best described in two stages (*a*) the stage of elevation, (*b*) the stage of depression.

(*a*) The Stage of Elevation.

Symptoms—Prodromata.—As a rule in such cases we obtain a history of a gradual change in character and disposition, that the patient has become "moody" and is sometimes elevated, at others depressed for short periods. Further, we are told that the periods of elevation have gradually become more frequent and pronounced until they have passed into the condition of continuous elevation in which we see the patient.

Physical Symptoms.—The majority of such patients appear healthy and by no means ill-nourished. The face is flushed, the eyes bright and, though unnaturally mobile, the expression is by no means unintelligent and lacks the confused appearance so common in cases of acute mania. The skin is moist and greasy, and, as a rule, gives off a most offensive odour. The temperature is as a rule febrile, generally from 100° to 102° F. at the commencement of an attack. The condition of the alimentary tract varies ; if the case be acute and be seen early, there may be gastric derangement, anæmia and complete distaste for both food and drink, but later on in the attack, especially if the patient has already suffered from this condition, the appetite becomes ravenous and the taste perverted, the patient craving for stimulants and condiments, and eating greedily things from which he would have turned with a shudder when in his proper mind. The pulse is of low tension and about normal in rate. The blood presents a hyperleucocytosis in the early stages, though not so marked an increase as in acute mania, the polymorphonuclear percentage however in a first attack may be well above 70. In recurrent attacks, as a rule, according to Dr. Bruce there is a fall both in the leucocytosis and in the polymorph percentage immediately before the onset of elevation. As the attack progresses the leucocytosis increases with the elevation, reaches a maximum at the height of the seizure, and then gradually falls to normal. The leucocytosis in such cases is however markedly irregular and tends to fall as the attack passes off and thus differs markedly from that of an attack of acute mania. The urine is diminished in amount, concentrated, highly coloured, deposits urates and occasionally has traces of sugar and albumen.

Subject-consciousness is diminished but sensibility to touch, heat and pain is markedly increased and the special senses are hyperacute. Superficial and deep reflexes are increased, as also the muscular tonus, while slight inco-ordination is present.

Mental Symptoms.—As already noted the mental condition is one of pure elevation without confusion and free from hallucinations or delusions. The hyperacute state of the special senses may however simulate hallucinations and this must be carefully looked for to avoid error in diagnosis. Self-control is lost but obsessions are rare in this condition, the diminished self-control being as a rule evidenced by extravagant but purposeful movement, noise and mischievous teasing conduct, such patients as a rule taking great delight in baiting some poor unfortunate fellow sufferer. Morality and decency are at a very low ebb in all these cases and the conduct and speech are oppressively lewd and coarse. The memory in a first attack may be diminished both for recent and past events, but when the attacks are recurrent the memory in the stage of elevation is phenomenal, long articles being repeated from the newspaper, and every small word or action of some fellow-patient during a previous attack being brought up and used to tease and annoy him. Such cases are extremely divertible, and, though their attention can readily be caught, it is impossible to hold it for any length of time owing to their great divertibility and prompt reaction to each and every passing stimulus. The speech, though irrelevant, is by no means incoherent, and the power of reading and writing remains, though the latter is often fantastic in character and crossed and underlined in a way only an insane person would think of doing. Insomnia is marked throughout the attack.

The duration of the elevation is very variable, from a few days to months, but whether long or short the patient's condition during an attack is one of extreme restlessness, both physically and mentally, he is extremely capricious and flighty, irritable and lacking in modesty, cleanliness and honesty. The restlessness gradually diminishes, sleep returns, the physical condition, which is affected by the elevation, improves and *pari passu* the patient returns by degrees to a condition of apparent sanity.

Diagnosis.—This stage of elevation has to be distinguished from acute mania and the acute stage of onset of many of the other acute insanities. The leucocytosis and the absence of confusion, hallucinations and delusions are the main points which enable us to distinguish this condition.

Treatment.—Rest in bed is essential, tending, as it does, to lessen the acute symptoms. Free purgation should be resorted to at the commencement of the case, and where gastric derangement is present, light diet given in small quantities at frequent intervals is necessary, but where a good appetite is present a full general dietary should be given to tide the patient over the acute symptoms with as little loss in physical condition as possible. In cases of extreme elevation and insomnia sedatives are indicated, and in my experience I have got best results from 10 minim doses of paraldehyde, or 10—15 grs. of sulphonal, given thrice daily. When the acute stage lessens, then exercise in the open air, tonics and carefully regulated employment are indicated.

Thyroid extract has been used in the treatment of this condition, but its applicability is very circumscribed as it is practically contraindicated when elevation is present, and is only occasionally of use in cutting short or aborting the stage of elevation when it can be anticipated and the drug administered before its advent. Even then however it must be exhibited with caution, as its excessive or prolonged use tends to increase and prolong the elevation.

Subcutaneous injections of turpentine have been used with the object of raising the leucocytosis and thus cutting short the attack, but the results so far have been disappointing, only a very small percentage showing any marked results.

Prognosis.—The immediate prognosis is good, recovery occurring in practically every case after a longer or shorter time. Recurrences however are inevitable and with each attack the prognosis becomes more unfavourable, as the tendency to pass into a condition of more or less secondary dementia becomes greater with every attack.

(*b*) The Stage of Depression.

Symptoms.—The stage of depression may either precede or follow the stage of elevation, and the *physical state* of the patient is markedly affected during this condition. There is marked gastric derangement, evidenced by anorexia, constipation and a furred flabby tongue. The heart is weak, and the pulse slow, irregular and feeble, but the arterial tension, as a rule, is high. The skin is greasy and offensive, and the extremities cyanosed and cold, and at times even œdematous in extreme cases tending to become stuporose. Hyperleucocytosis is nearly always present, but there is never any marked rise in the polymorphonuclear percentage. Sensibility to touch, heat and pain is unaffected, but the special senses are less acute than is normally the case.

Mentally.—The condition is one of pure apathy and depression, without confusion or the presence of hallucinations and delusions. In some cases, where the depression follows after a stage of elevation, the apathy and depression are so marked after the restlessness and noise that one is almost led to think the condition one of secondary dementia.

As with the stage of elevation, so here the recovery is gradual and *pari passu* with the physical improvement.

Diagnosis.—The absence of confusion and of hallucinations and delusions enables us to distinguish this stage of folie circulaire from acute and excited melancholia.

Treatment.—Rest in bed and a light nourishing diet are absolutely essential here. For constipation large saline enemata are of the utmost use and should be given about twice a week. The enemata probably help also in removing more toxic material from the bowel than would be done by ordinary purgatives, and in addition a certain amount must be absorbed and thus the excretion of toxines by the skin and kidneys may be aided. For insomnia paraldehyde ʒii is invaluable, if a hot glass of milk and a hot bath at bed time prove useless, though they should undoubtedly be given a good trial before we resort to drugs.

Prognosis.—The prognosis here is the same as for the stage of elevation (q. v.).

KATATONIA.

This condition was first described by Kahlbaum in 1874, and derives its name from the muscular rigidity which is one of its characteristic symptoms. More recently Kræpelin has described it as one of the three varieties of what he terms "Dementia Præcox" (hebephrenia and paranoia being the two other varieties), and though I consider this classification unsound, grouping, as it does, three distinct and separate diseases under one head, as varieties of one condition, Kraepelin's description of this condition is undoubtedly the more scientific of the two.

Definition.—Katatonia may be defined as an acute toxic disease, with a definite course and onset, characterised by a prodromal period leading gradually to an acute period of onset marked by mental confusion, aural hallucinations, paroxysms of fear or anger, obsessions, a katatonic spasm of the muscles and a marked hyperleucocytosis indicating an acute toxæmia. In the second stage a condition of stupor, without loss of consciousness, supervenes, which is characterised by marked resistiveness to passive movements and is followed as a rule by the third stage of excitement.

Ætiology.—This condition is equally common among Europeans, Eurasians and natives of India. As a rule, it commences in adolescence and so far as my experience in India goes seems more common among males ; this, however, may be due to the habits of the Indian and the extreme reluctance with which he sends any of his women to an institution, for in Europe the incidence falls more heavily on females. Hereditary taint is present in the large majority of such cases, but any condition tending to lower the vitality and resistance to infective conditions renders the person liable to this disease.

Symptoms.—(*a*) PRODROMATA.—In every case one elicits a history of insidious onset with gradual loss of energy and failure of nutrition. Hallucinations of hearing are, as a rule, the first signs of mental aberration noted and sooner or later give rise to delusions, obsessions and complete loss of self-control. It is at this point the patients are usually sent to an asylum, and by far the majority are thin and badly nourished by the time we receive them.

(*b*) ACUTE STAGE OF ONSET—**Physical Symptoms.**—Gastric derangement, evidenced by anorexia and occasional nausea and vomiting, is invariably present in such cases. The arterial tension rises as the symptoms become more acute, and the heart becomes irritable and its action rapid and irregular. The skin is moist and greasy, and drenching perspirations occur frequently, while blotchy pustular rashes are seen in many cases. There is a moderate hyperleucocytosis, and an increase in the polymorph and hyaline elements throughout this stage, and just prior to the onset of the stage of stupor there is a sudden rise in the leucocytosis due mainly to an increase in the polymorphonuclear elements. Sensibility to touch, heat and pain is diminished, and the senses of taste and smell are often completely perverted, but, so far as can be ascertained, the senses of sight and hearing react normally to outward impressions, though auditory, and occasionally visual, hallucinations are seen in this stage. The pupils are, as a rule, dilated and react sluggishly to light, and the organic reflexes are deranged, such patients as a rule, being wet and dirty, and requiring constant attention. The superficial and deep reflexes are invariably exaggerated, while the voluntary muscles are liable to pass into fits of rigidity or "katatonic spasm" which may last from a few minutes to a few hours. Insomnia is invariably present to a varying extent. The temperature in these cases is irregular, at times paradoxical, but rarely markedly febrile during the acute stage of onset, though a distinct febrile attack invariably ushers in the stage of stupor.

Mental Symptoms.—In this stage of the disease the mental condition is essentially one of confusion, while vivid and terrifying auditory hallucinations affect the conduct and frequently lead to paroxysms of terror during which the patient may make frantic attempts to hide from his imaginary enemies, or, finding attempts at concealment of no avail, may attempt to place himself beyond their power by committing suicide. In the intervals between paroxysms the patient may lie for hours, with closed eyes, apparently oblivious to all that happens around him or, in other cases, there may be brief periods of apparent sanity, in which however a certain amount of confusion still remains and there is a lack of the faculty of attention and of memory for recent events.

Diagnosis.—The history of onset, the results of a blood examination, the temperature and the marked state of mental confusion with auditory hallucinations are our main points in diagnosing this condition.

Treatment.—Rest in bed with a light nourishing dietary are essential in this stage. Nourishment should be given frequently and in small quantity at a time, and the patient should invariably have nourishment administered during the night. Normal saline solution administered either subcutaneously or per rectum seems in some cases to give a certain amount of relief and even to induce sleep at times. If insomnia be trying, the effects of a hot bath and a hot glass of milk at bed-time should be tried, and if these fail then recourse must be had to drugs and of these I prefer large doses of paraldehyde ʒiii to ʒiv administered every third night, though I have at times had good results from sulphonal grs. x combined with potassium bromide grs. xxx.

Prognosis.—The acute stage terminates as a rule, after 4—6 weeks, in a distinct febrile attack which ushers in the stage of stupor. Death however may occur during this stage from exhaustion or from an exceptionally virulent toxæmia.

(c) Stage of Stupor.

This stage of the disease occurs, as a rule, immediately after the febrile attack already noted as terminating the acute stage of the malady. In some cases however the febrile attack may be wanting and the stage of stupor then occurs after the high leucocytosis which terminates the preceding stage.

Physical Symptoms.—Gastric derangement is still marked throughout this stage and constipation is often most troublesome. The arterial tension falls below normal and the cardiac action is weak and slow. Blood examination reveals a persistent hyperleucocytosis with a high lymphocyte percentage and at times a transient eosinophilia. The extremities are cyanosed and cold, and the feet and hands are often œdematous. The skin is greasy and gives off a close offensive odour and at times a fine branny desquamation occurs. The temperature as a rule is subnormal, with occasional sudden rises to 100°—101°F. The organic reflexes are as a rule ignored, and retention of urine and fæces is therefore to be constantly looked for and treated. The superficial reflexes are active, but the deep reflexes cannot be elicited on account of the spasmodic muscular resistance caused by any attempt at passive movement. The sensibility and special senses, owing to the condition of the patient, cannot be satisfactorily tested during this stage, but, as the patient is fully aware of all that goes on around him, the probability is that the special senses at least are quite active. The power to sleep returns during this stage and somnolence is often excessive, the patient being always drowsy and heavy.

Mental Symptoms.—The mental condition during this stage of the disease is one of semi-conscious stupor. Hallucinations, both visual and auditory, complicate the condition and give rise to various delusions. Obsessions, attitudinising, mutism, rhythmical movements and repetitions of words, letters and numbers, sudden outbursts of excitement, and obstinate resistance to any attempts at movement or assistance in feeding and dressing are invariably present in a more or less marked degree in every case. Masturbation is very common in such conditions, but seems to partake more of the character of an automatic movement than of eroticism. Attempts at suicide or homicide occasionally occur and must always be carefully guarded against; they are due as a rule to sudden impulses and originate probably in some hallucination or delusion.

Diagnosis.—The condition of semi-conscious stupor with fixed attitudes and an extreme state of negativism are characteristic of this stage and when seen form an unmistakable picture.

Treatment.—The stage of katatonic stupor is a most trying one for the alienist to treat. Fresh air, tonics, a full dietary and patience are one and all essential for a successful issue. Beyond these and the observance of ordinary hygienic measures nothing can be done. Above all no attempt must be made to force the patient more than is absolutely necessary, for no good but only harm can accrue thereby, thus exercise must only be voluntary on the part of the patient and no attempt be made to force him to it. When the patient shows signs of recovery hot baths with a little mustard in them may hasten the process, but caution must be exercised in their use and a raised temperature or unduly increased rate or tension of pulse indicates their immediate suspension.

Prognosis.—The stage of stupor is of uncertain duration and may last from a few weeks to a few years. In favourable cases, which recover without passing into a stage of excitement, the leucocytosis remains high and the polymorphonuclear percentage rarely falls much below 60%, and conversely a leucocytosis much below 10,000 and a polymorphonuclear percentage of 50 or less, occurring early in the stage of stupor, is a bad prognostic symptom. Where the stupor is of long duration the prognosis is always bad.

(*d*). THE STAGE OF EXCITEMENT.—This as a rule occurs immediately after the stage of stupor, though occasionally there is an apparent recovery from the stage of stupor and then the patient relapses after even two or three years. In some very exceptional cases however recovery seems to follow on after the stage of stupor and no subsequent relapse occurs, but such an event is rare and should never be spoken of too hopefully.

Physical Symptoms.—The excitement in this stage is by no means continuous but comes on in bursts between which there are remissions to apparent sanity. Gastric derangement is much less marked and the cardiac functions approximate more closely to the normal. There is still a tendency to fall into fixed attitudes or rhythmical movements, such as "doing sentry-go," stereotyped movements of the hands and irregular action of the facial muscles. Between the bursts of excitement however the patient is comparatively quiet and shows no marked symptom of mental derangement.

Mental Symptoms.—Confusion is still present to a certain extent in this stage though much less marked than in the stage of stupor. Memory, both past and present, is impaired and the power of attention diminished, the patient in fact showing all the signs of a more or less marked secondary dementia, which is only to be expected after the severe mental attacks he has already come through. Hallucinations and delusions are markedly pronounced in these cases and are very liable to affect the conduct, so that patients in this stage of the disease require constant care and supervision.

Diagnosis.—Without a history of the previous stage of stupor such cases are practically impossible to diagnose with certainty, and hence arises one of our main difficulties in asylum diagnosis in India for, as a rule, the information received with cases is most meagre.

Treatment.—A full nourishing dietary with tonics, especially iron and quinine, is indicated during this stage. If the excitement be so intense and prolonged that the patient becomes exhausted, then rest in bed becomes necessary and sedatives are essential. In such cases sulphonal grs. x, thrice daily is most useful, but I have also had good result at times from a combination of Tr. Hyoscyamus with Tr. Cannabis Indicæ.

Prognosis.—The older the patient the less tendency there is for the disease to terminate in marked dementia, but as a rule some mental enfeeblement invariably remains. In adolescent cases the outlook is very bad and complete recovery rarely, if ever, occurs. (As a rule a little over 20% make complete recoveries, 20% partial recoveries with a certain amount of dementia, and the remaining 60% remain in a state of chronic irritable dementia till death occurs.)

HEBEPHRENIA.

This term was first applied, by Kahlbaum or Hecker, to certain pathological mental disturbances which occur in puberty or early adult life. Kræpelin has included this condition, as already mentioned, in his description of Dementia Præcox and the error thus entailed has been already discussed. It is only in recent years that this malady has begun to be recognised in Great Britain as a separate disease, Clouston grouping it among the insanities of adolescence, Macpherson wholly ignoring it and many other authors denying its existence. Gradually, however, it has forced itself upon the medical world and now, instead of regarding the symptoms as due to premature brain involution leading ultimately to dementia, the majority of alienists recognise it as a distinct entity.

Definition.—Briefly it may be defined as a disease of adolescence in which the symptoms, both physical and mental, run a subacute but definite course and in which the symptom of hyperleucocytosis is so frequently met with as to justify its inclusion among Insanities due to Bacterial Toxæmias.

Ætiology.—This disease is essentially an affection of early adolescence and I have never seen a case which began its course in adult life. It affects alike Europeans, Eurasians and natives of India. In Europe females are more frequently affected than males, and having regard to the customs and prejudices of the native and the possibility of treating such cases at home, I am convinced in my own mind that the same holds good out here, for though among natives asylum statistics might lead us to think otherwise, yet among Europeans and Eurasians in Asylums in India, undoubtedly a larger percentage of females is affected by this condition than is the case with the males.

Hereditary predisposition is a marked ætiological factor in this disease, Kahlbaum's statistics showing it to be present in over 50% of cases.

The precise cause of this condition is as yet unknown. So far no evidences of metabolic toxæmia have been found and the frequency with which hyperleucocytosis is seen in these cases leads Dr. Bruce to enter it among insanities due to bacterial toxæmias, and I feel I cannot do better than follow his example.

Symptoms—Prodromata.—The onset of this condition is invariably gradual and insidious, the patient, who, as a child, was probably intelligent and precocious, changing in character, losing the power of sustained attention and the capacity for work, and showing peculiarities in conduct varying from mere eccentricities up to undoubted mental derangement. As a rule such cases hate society and lead a friendless existence, wandering aimlessly about, unable to settle to any work or amusement, and more often than not becoming dissolute or mischievous. Such cases, as a rule, are given to masturbation, and may often be seen in a solitary corner, where they fancy they are unperceived, giggling and muttering to themselves and indulging in this disgusting habit.

During this insidious onset the patient's friends and relatives are very apt to misunderstand matters and resort either to spiritual exhortation or to physical repression for its cure, with the result that the condition becomes worse instead of better, as diminished self-control renders the patient liable to outbursts of irritability or violence with little or no provocation, and it is at this stage that the patients are usually placed under medical care.

Physical Symptoms.—Arrest of physical developement is a striking feature in all cases, patients of twenty-five or twenty-six years of age looking immature and about fifteen or sixteen years old or even less, and this abnormally youthful appearance lasts throughout life. The expression of the face is dull, heavy and furtive. Movements are awkward and there is marked disinclination for active exercise, such patients being as a rule lethargic and preferring to sit idle all day long. Among Indians such cases are frequently enormously stout, and at times I have seen cases where there was no marked arrest of physical developement. The temperature, on the whole, remains practically normal, though every now and then during an exacerbation, when the patient becomes restless and sleepless, the thermometer in the evening may, for a week or so, register about 100°F.

The pulse is normal in rate and tension, as a rule, except during the exacerbations when it tends to become faster and irregular. Dr. Bruce states that a small hyperleucocytosis of 12,000—14,000 per c.m.m. is as a rule present, but in some cases this is greatly increased, the hyalines and large lymphocytes being apparently most implicated in the rise, the polymorphonuclear cells remaining about their normal percentage.

Amenorrhœa is constantly present among women, and both sexes are addicted to masturbation when suffering from this condition.

Sensibility to touch, heat and pain is unaffected, and the special senses too seem normal.

The organic reflexes are under control, the superficial and deep reflexes are normal, and there is no paralysis or diminished co-ordination of the voluntary muscles.

Mental Symptoms.—The outstanding mental symptom in such cases is the gradually progressive dementia which overtakes the patient. Affection for relatives and friends is lost, the faculty of attention and *pari passu* the capability for work is diminished, the power of volition is gone, and such cases sit idly day after day contented with doing nothing, and, so far as one can see, not even troubling themselves to think. Memory though fair for recent events during the earlier stages becomes markedly impaired as the disease progresses. Speech is markedly affected, in the earlier stages it is hesitating and jerky, and, as the disease advances, this function becomes more and more impaired till finally all power is practically gone and the patient remains mute and silent, or, after much interrogation, simply jerks out parrot-like one or two phrases, no matter what question may have been put to him. Confusion is never markedly present in such cases and the mood is variable, patients being perhaps one day dull and suspicious and next day irritable. Neither hallucinations nor delusions are common in this malady, and the former when present are usually hallucinations of hearing and may lead to obsessions, impulsive acts and general restlessness. Sleep is invariably abolished during the periods of exacerbation, and in some cases a curious condition may be noticed, the patient sleeping one night, being wakeful for the next one or two, and then sleeping again on the second or third night.

Diagnosis.—The previous history of the case, the hesitating jerky speech, the gradual progressive dementia, and last, but not least, the retarded developement of the patient are what we must look for to help us in our diagnosis of such cases.

Treatment.—The treatment of such cases can, until more is known as to its cause and origin, be on merely general lines. During the acute exacerbations rest in bed may be necessary, but otherwise routine discipline, light regular work when possible, and a non-stimulating fattening diet produce the best results. In cases where sleep is deranged I have found sulphonal invaluable in breaking the periodicity and inducing a normal "sleep habit."

Prognosis.—This as a rule is indicated to a certain extent by the developement of the patient, recovery being most likely to occur where developement is fuller, and in those few cases which do recover there is invariably a marked improvement in developement coincident with the abatement of the mental symptoms. In any case, however, the prognosis is by no means favourable. Kræpelin's statistics in Europe show a recovery rate of about 5 per cent. and about 15% remain partially demented, though so far recovered as to be able to live at home, but the remainder pass into a condition of hopeless dementia. My little knowledge of such cases in India leads me to believe that the outlook here is much less hopeful even than the above, but statistics on this condition are hard to find, and, allowing for cases treated at home, possibly the prognosis may be much the same out here.

CHAPTER XIV

INSANITIES OF TOXIC ORIGIN—(*contd.*)

Group III. Insanities due to Drug and Alcoholic Toxines.

INSANITY DUE TO THE ABUSE OF CANNABIS INDICA.

I have given this drug first place in its class as it is the most common in use among the natives in India, in one or other of its forms, and is one of the most frequent causes of the insanity in asylums. "Indian Hemp," as it is commonly called, is cultivated largely throughout India and Central Asia and especially in the hilly country of Northern India. In fact in these districts it may be found growing wild and apparently flourishing well at the commencement of the hot weather.

It is used in various forms and many are the names applied to it in different districts. The four main preparations however are (*a*) Ganjah or ganga, (*b*) bhang, (*c*) charas, (*d*) haschisch.

(*a*) *Ganjah* is the dried flowering tops, consisting of stem, leaves and flowers, of the cultivated female plants, which, having been unable to set seeds freely, become coated with resin. It is the form most commonly used in Bengal for smoking, and is as a rule mixed with tobacco, its retail price being about Rs. 2 a seer (2lbs.)

(*b*) *Bhang* is a mixture of the dried leaves and capsule. It is the cheapest form of the drug, and is made into various decoctions. It is the form in which Sikhs commonly take the drug. It costs ordinarily about 8 annas per seer.

(*c*) *Charas* is the resinous exudate, obtained by rubbing the cut female heads, which have been previously dried for twenty-four hours, between the hands, and then scraping off the resin which adheres to the hands. It is the most concentrated and at the same time the most expensive form of the drug, costing about Rs. 35 per seer. It is used either mixed with tobacco for smoking or is swallowed whole in pillular form.

(*d*) *Haschisch* is a confection prepared from *charas* and more common in Arabia than in India.

In addition to the above many local beverages and decoctions exist, but the names of these are as legion as the preparations themselves, and it is useless to cumber the brain with them.

Ætiology.—It is quite a common habit among the general population to use a certain amount of *bhang* in the hot weather as a "cooling drink," and taken thus in small quantity and in weak solution it is quite harmless. When, however, any form of the drug is taken in large quantity, or for long continued periods, the results are disastrous, as is apparent in those who resort to it as a form of dissipation and indulge in it to a gradually increasing extent.

It is but seldom that any native, except perhaps a *faquir*, indulges in any form of the drug by himself. Thus it is a common custom among Sikhs to have one large vessel containing *bhang* in their temples or at their festivities, and from this all those present help themselves, and when among other castes the drug is smoked it is almost invariably enjoyed in company, one man pulling at the *chillum* till he becomes dazed and then passing it on to his neighbour.

Many and various are the reasons I have heard given for the commencement of the habit, some say that it is to obtain a feeling of restfulness, others that it aids digestion, while some affirm, after close questioning, that they use it on account of its powers as an aphrodisiac, or have acquired the habit from associating with *faquirs.* In this connection it is interesting to note that *faquirs*, as a rule, are addicted to the use, or shall we say abuse, of *charas*, and justify this by stating that while *bhang* and *ganjah* are undoubted aphrodisiacs *charas* on the contrary is an aphrodisiac, and that it is for this reason they take it. Whether this be so or not, it is however an undoubted fact that the general population condones this indulgence of the *faquir* and his disciples, though they regard the other classes of its consumers, and rightly too, as dissipated loafers who have taken to the drug from idleness and viciousness.

Though so generally in use among the natives only a very small number are seriously addicted to the drug, about ·5 per cent. according to the report of the Commission held on it in 1894, and its evil effects can be imagined when fully 30% of the male inmates of the Agra Asylum, the cause of whose insanity can be elicited, are said to have been addicted to this habit.

Many natives affirm that this habit has a great advantage over indulgence in opium, alcohol or even tobacco, because it can be given up at any time without difficulty. To a certain extent this is correct, as I have noticed time and again that sudden stoppage of the drug, even against the will of the patient, is productive of none of the physical effects which occur after sudden stoppage of other drugs, such as opium, etc. It is, however, an undoubted fact that excessive indulgence in any form of the drug does produce a violent craving for it, and that the amount taken is gradually increased. Apart from the physical effects too, such as anorexia, debility and muscular tremors, there is in those addicted to the abuse of the drug a general moral deterioration, very similar to that seen in those who indulge to excess in opium or alcohol, such people hesitating at nothing to obtain the drug and spending their last pie on it rather than on food or clothing for their families.

Cases of insanity assigned to this cause show, both from the mental and physical aspect, a striking uniformity of symptoms, a uniformity indeed so striking that it at once precludes any possibility of error in the cause assigned.

Symptoms.—The description of the effects of over-indulgence in this drug is best divided into two groups :—

(*a*) Acute cases, under which we may class the simple intoxication, produced by a large dose of the drug in persons unused to it, and the transitory mania which often follows on after such intoxication.

(*b*) Chronic cases, under which head we may describe the effects of the drug on those who are well accustomed to it and on whom the results are more marked and longer in duration.

(*a*) ACUTE CASES.

1. Acute Intoxication—**Physical Symptoms**. In cases where a large dose has been taken by one unused to the drug a condition of intoxication is produced. The patient's eyes are bloodshot and the pupils dilated. General sensibility is markedly diminished and there is a great inclination for muscular activity and a marked tendency to perform acts of violence with a complete disregard of the consequences, and, as already noted in a previous chapter, cases of "running amuck" are frequently seen in this condition of intoxication.

Mental Symptoms.—The first effects of a large dose is a feeling of giddiness, which gradually wears off and is replaced by a condition of ecstacy or excitement with which there is a marked degree of confusion. Delusions and hallucinations, both visual and auditory, flit through the patient's mind in rapid succession keeping him entranced with delight, and by their rapid passage seeming to prolong time. This condition generally passes into a deep sleep from which the patients awake to find that, but for the initial symptoms, they have no memory of anything that has occurred. This lapse of memory is very typical of intoxication from this drug and occurs also after the transitory maniacal attacks which sometimes follow on the acute intoxication. The forgetfulness may last for some weeks after all other symptoms of intoxication have departed.

Treatment.—In a case of acute intoxication, when perhaps insensibility is setting in, the only remedy is prompt and complete evacuation of the stomach and bowels and the administration of stimulants. Vinegar, acetic, citric and tartaric acids have been recommended as antidotes. The body should be kept warm by blankets and hot bottles.

A fact well worth remembering is that coffee, tea and cocoa are said to increase the action of the drug and should never be used in such cases.

2. Transitory condition of Excitement.—This condition of acute maniacal symptoms as a rule follows after an acute intoxication in one addicted to the chronic abuse of the drug. It is an important one from a medico-legal point of view, for there is no condition in which acts of reckless violence and brutality are more liable to be committed, and, taking Mr. Justice Stephen's definition of responsibility into consideration, it is apparently nothing but justice to hold such cases responsible for acts which were committed during a period of intoxication which they knowingly and willingly entered. It is the commonest asylum form of mental conditions due to Cannabis Indica and is generally of short duration, the symptoms ceasing so soon as the supply of the drug is stopped.

Physical Symptoms.—The temperature is as a rule slightly febrile, the eyes bloodshot, the horizontal ciliary branches being chiefly affected, and the pupils dilated and the face flushed, with an expression of demoniacal excitement.

Mental Symptoms.—The mental condition is one of intense excitement and confusion. The patients are intensely noisy and restless, and become irritated at the slightest attempt to control them. Hallucinations of sight and hearing are especially characteristic of this condition, and partake as a rule of a sensual character, lovely females being said to visit the patients at night and converse with them, etc., etc. These symptoms as a rule subside quickly once the supply of the drug is stopped, and are followed by complete oblivion to all that happened during the period of excitement.

Diagnosis.—The history of the case, the marked confusion, and above all the recklessness and violence of the patient are absolutely unmistakeable, and form a picture which once seen can never be forgotten.

Treatment.—Prompt and complete removal of the drug, with non-stimulating nourishing diet, and careful supervision to prevent acts of violence as a rule suffice in such cases. At times sedatives may be necessary, and on such occasions I have got good results from paraldehyde ʒiii—ʒiv every second day, or sulphonal grs. x morning and evening, but, as a rule, after a day or two of acute excitement the symptoms gradually subside and no further trouble is experienced in treating the case.

Prognosis.—The prognosis in this condition is invariably most hopeful, such cases recovering rapidly and perfectly once the drug is completely removed from them. It is as well, however, to keep them under treatment for as long as possible to make sure of their complete recovery from the habit, for if they again take to the drug when discharged relapses are sure to ensue.

(*b*) CHRONIC CASES.

These occur in those much addicted to the drug, and generally as a result of a rapid increase in the amount of the drug consumed or of a too frequent indulgence in it.

Symptoms.—The symptoms are practically identical with the acute mania already described, but recovery is much slower as a rule.

Prognosis.—The majority of such cases recover after a time, but a certain number continue in a state of chronic excitement until death, while a still smaller number relapse into a condition of dementia in which they ultimately die.

INSANITY DUE TO THE ABUSE OF ALCOHOL.

There is no more common exciting cause of insanity among Europeans and Eurasians as a whole than alcohol, for though Cannabis Indica stands pre-eminent in India as an exciting cause among Indians, yet alcohol is freely used by Europeans and Eurasians, and, besides its direct results on the individual, leaves its taint upon the offspring, rendering them specially prone to intemperance, epilepsy, idiocy and insanity. The crude liquor too so commonly seen in the bazaars, and in which certain classes of natives and Eurasians indulge freely, is specially noxious and produces much more disastrous results than the matured imported liquors.

The effects of alcohol vary greatly, not only between individuals but between races, and various explanations have been brought forward for this. The form of liquor indulged in has, and undoubtedly with some reason, been brought forward as an explanation by some, while others again say that a species of "alcoholic immunity" is produced in races who have drunk hard for centuries, and the proof of this is that most primitive races are extremely intolerant of liquor and, unless the supply be stopped, it may even threaten the very existence of such races. Other points than these however have probably more to do with the matter. Thus the effects of alcohol are invariably greater upon those sprung from neurotic stock, and by far the majority of habitual inebriates will on enquiry be found to have a tainted heredity. In fact just as an alcoholic parent may beget an epileptic or an idiot, so a parent who is of weak nervous stability, an epileptic, etc., etc., may beget offspring who readily fall into alcoholic habits, and the close connection between this habit and the neuroses cannot be too strongly brought forward.

A very small amount of alcohol too, rapidly produces a most pernicious effect on persons who have previously suffered from head injuries or sunstroke, as well as on epileptics who have at any time suffered from insanity.

Besides its effects on the nervous system we must also remember its effects on the body generally, and that by lowering the general resistance to infection by bacterial organisms it must of necessity be a strong predisposing factor to most of the insanities due to bacterial toxæmias.

In fact, as Craig ably puts it, "alcoholism is so far-reaching in its results that in the individual we find a progressive tendency to mental and bodily deterioration and a lowered resistance to bodily disease; in the offspring a proneness to idiocy, epilepsy and criminality; and in the race a higher disease rate, a higher mortality rate, and a lowered birth rate."

Ætiology.—A neurotic inheritance is by far the most important factor. Some writers go so far as to state that an acquired taint is not transmitted to the offspring, but this certainly does not apply to alcoholism, and I know of several families where the tendency has been transmitted through three or four generations.

Habit is also an important factor in this condition, many persons first taking the drug from social or business reasons, and then gradually increasing the amount till they find themselves slaves to a habit from which they cannot free themselves.

Others again resort to alcohol to stimulate a worn out brain and body to fresh exertion, instead of restoring them by the rest and nourishment they require, with the inevitable result that a mental breakdown sooner or later occurs and is probably complicated by the alcohol taken to stave it off.

In this connection it must be remembered that alcoholism may be but one of the early symptoms of an attack of one of the acute insanities, or may be the sole remnant of a previous attack and due to the diminished self-control resulting therefrom.

Varieties.—As with Cannabis Indica, so with alcohol, we meet with both acute and chronic intoxications.

In the former conditions the symptoms are due wholly to the direct action of the poison on the nervous centres, but in the latter they are often due to structural alterations in the cerebral blood-vessels and nervous elements.

Roughly they may be classified into (*a*) Acute Intoxication. (*b*) Delirium Tremens. (*c*) Mania à potu. (*d*) Chronic alcoholic insanity. (*e*) Dipsomania.

(*a*) Acute Intoxication.

Physical Symptoms.—These vary greatly with the individual, but roughly they may be classified into two groups. In the first of these sickness and subsequent gastritis are the main symptoms, while in the second motor inco-ordination and subsequent severe headache are most prominent.

Mental Symptoms.—Alcohol tends to exaggerate the normal temperament, the weak-minded person becoming foolish, the morose man tending to weep or become sullen, and the excitable individual becoming merry and exalted under its influence. Many and varied, however, are the types of mental derangement associated with this condition, from stupor and extreme mental confusion to a state of wild excitement, and as the disturbance is, as a rule, over in a few hours there is but little need to cumber such a book as this with them. It is as well to note, however, that occasionally the mental disorder may last for days or even weeks, and in some cases epileptic convulsions may occur.

Treatment.—An emetic and forcible confinement in bed is all that is required in such cases.

(b) Delirium Tremens.

This condition may arise in several ways. It may be the result of an excessive amount of alcohol consumed in a comparatively short space of time, or on the contrary the sudden suspension of the drug may suffice to originate an attack, or it may occur after an injury or shock, or complicate an illness, such as typhoid or pneumonia.

Physical Symptoms.—Gastric derangement is the most marked physical symptom of this condition, and is evidenced by anorexia, a furred tremulous tongue, constipation and gastric pain and uneasiness with occasional vomiting. The skin is, as a rule, moist, and drenching perspiration may occur at times, while the temperature rarely rises above 100° F. Muscular tremors are marked and the speech is often affected thereby, while in a few cases epileptic convulsions may occur. Sleeplessness is invariably met with in such cases, and when marked is of great prognostic import. There is nearly always a moderate hyperleucocytosis in such cases.

Mental Symptoms.—The onset is not as a rule sudden, as is popularly supposed, but is preceded by a condition of neuro-muscular irritability. The patient is excited and impulsive, becomes timid, suspicious and restless and is generally very irritable. Night as a rule intensifies this condition and the patient passes the hours of darkness in an agony of terror, misinterpreting every sound and haunted by hallucinations both of sight and hearing. Animals and insects crawl around and on his bed, while devils torment and jeer at him, and it is characteristic of this condition that the hallucinations are invariably of a terrifying, awe-inspiring kind. As the case progresses these hallucinations appear by day as well as by night, and the patient spends the hours in one continuous agony of fear.

In very rare cases for a few brief hours these terrifying phantoms disappear and the patient passes into a condition of exaltation with grandiose delusions as to his own position and importance, but soon this condition vanishes and the patient returns to his former state of terror. Where this condition is seen the case, as a rule, terminates in complete dementia. In such cases cognition is as a rule poor, and memory, though fair for remote events, fails altogether when recent events are brought forward for discussion. Attention is wholly self-centred and objective, and such patients spend the time wrapt up in themselves and their hallucinations and delusions. Suicide is often attempted in these cases, and one has to be constantly on one's guard against it.

Diagnosis.—Acute mania is the chief condition likely to be confused with this, and the history and the somatic symptoms, along with the character of the hallucinations are our chief diagnostic aids.

Treatment.—Rest in bed and frequent feeding with small quantities of fluid food, preferably milk and soda, are essential in all cases. In the very early stages a full dose of chloral and bromide may produce sleep and cut short the attack, but otherwise hypnotics must be used with the greatest caution and paraldehyde is especially contraindicated as it seems rather to increase the excitement. Insomnia is best treated by hot baths, and the effects of these may be increased by hot draughts of milk and cold applications to the head. If there is a tendency to collapse, hypodermics of strychnine and warm saline enemata are invaluable. All such cases require careful supervision and control as there is constant danger of suicide and impulsive acts.

Prognosis.—Recovery is in the majority of cases complete and occurs in from 6—10 days, but one attack renders the patient more liable to subsequent ones. Where the course of the disease is prolonged there are always certain dangers ahead, thus the patient may pass into a condition of stupor and coma and ultimately die (about 5%); the hallucinations and delusions may persist after the subsidence of the other symptoms; a certain degree of dementia may remain after the attack; or lastly the condition may pass into one of ordinary acute mania.

(c) Mania a potu.

This is another but less common form of acute alcoholism, but a knowledge of it is important to the medical practitioner from a medico-legal point of view.

Ætiology.—There is usually in these cases a marked hereditary taint, and in many cases quite small doses of alcohol suffice to produce this condition.

Physical Symptoms.—The general health in such cases is as a rule good, and there is no appearance of illness which is so markedly present in delirium tremens. Insomnia is practically the only physical derangement, and a very trying one it is, and sleep has constantly to be produced by artificial means. The leucocytosis is as a rule fairly normal.

Mental Symptoms.—The condition here is one of intense mental and motor excitement, sudden in onset and extreme in violence, homicidal attacks being by no means infrequent. Such cases are invariably exalted, boastful and extravagant. Loss of self-control is evidenced by extreme irritability and sudden impulsive acts of violence. Hallucinations are by no means necessary concomitants of this condition, nor is confusion ever present to any marked extent.

Diagnosis.—This is as a rule easy when a clear history of the case is obtainable. The main conditions to be distinguished are other forms of excitement, epileptic furor, and the acute maniacal state which at times ushers in General Paralysis of the Insane.

Treatment.—The question of certification and treatment in an asylum is always one of extreme difficulty in these cases. The extreme violence and excitement renders them most difficult, in fact dangerous, to treat at home, but on the other hand when placed on proper treatment recovery is rapid as a rule, and the patient and his relatives are apt to blame the medical man for having unnecessarily confined him in an asylum and brought the blight thereof on the family. In such cases therefore a family conclave to decide the treatment to be adopted is always advisable, and thereat the probable course and dangers of the illness should be fully explained to the relatives, and it should be left to them to decide, in consultation, what line of treatment is to be adopted.

Rest in bed is essential, as also a full nourishing diet, and in these cases the alcohol may be withdrawn at once.

Restlessness, excitement and insomnia call for the administration of hypnotics, but these must be given sparingly and with caution to avoid the commencement of a drug habit. The bowels require constant attention as constipation is apt to be troublesome, and retention of urine has also at times to be guarded against.

Prognosis.—Rapid recovery is the rule in these cases, and once the patient is placed under proper care and treatment improvement progresses rapidly. Four to six weeks is the average duration of this condition, and I know of one or two cases where recovery occurred in a few days.

(*d*) Chronic Alcoholic Insanity.

Ætiology.—This form of intoxication arises as the result of steady drinking for months or even years. The symptoms vary with the individual, thus in one person the condition may be one of steadily progressive dementia, in others a condition of stupor or confusion may be present, others again may reveal a condition resembling delusional insanity, while in some cases a condition closely akin to General Paralysis of the Insane may be present.

Physical Symptoms.—These vary greatly with the individual. As a rule the patient has a bloated unhealthy appearance and a heavy, morose and vacant expression. The eyes are bloodshot and may be slightly jaundiced, and the small subcutaneous veins of the face are congested.

Gastric derangements are invariable concomitants of this condition, and reveal themselves by anorexia, pain and discomfort after taking food, constipation or diarrhœa, and emesis which is, as a rule, most frequent in the mornings.

The heart's action is irregular and weak, the arterial tension low and valvular lesions are common in such cases. Blood examination never reveals a hyperleucocytosis in this condition.

Albumen and sugar are frequently present in the urine, and carbuncles and boils are often met with and cause trouble.

There is general loss of muscular tonus, speech is blurred and defective due to tremors of the lips and tongue, and tremors, twitchings and cramps may affect any part of the muscular system, twitching of the supraorbital muscles being especially characteristic of alcoholic intoxications.

The gait is uncertain and hesitating, and the knee-jerks are at times absent, but may be exaggerated or unequal.

Peripheral neuritis may complicate this condition, in which case the patient may be unable to walk and may lose all control of his sphincters.

The physical and mental failure follows the ordinary course of events, the most recently acquired and most finely developed movements and faculties disappearing first.

The pupils are markedly unequal in many cases, and in a small number of patients the reaction to light may be markedly impaired, though some authorities deny this, and, if present, say it is due to some intercurrent disease.

Sensibility to touch, heat and pain may be variously affected, but hypersensibility to pain is a very common symptom.

Perversions of the special senses are common and frequently give rise to hallucinations and delusions.

Weight falls rapidly as a rule and the various organs are all more or less impaired in their functions.

Mental Symptoms.—The delusional type is by far the most common form of this disease. The delusions arise in practically every case from hallucinations originating in the perverted sensibility, both general and special, which gives rise to suspicions of poisoning, mesmerism, electricity, etc., and soon the patient weaves out a wonderful romance as to who his persecutors are, their reasons for persecuting him, and the means they employ.

The emotional state varies in such patients. Usually a condition of depression prevails, but outbursts of excitement may occur, in which violent attacks may be made upon the supposed persecutors.

Memory is invariably affected in these cases, recent memory being most affected at first, the amnesia gradually extending to more remote events as the disease progresses, and curiously enough with this loss of memory there is in most cases a concomitant loss of the craving for drink.

Suspicion is a common factor in all cases of alcoholic toxæmia and gives rise to delusions of persecution, the patient believing his wife unfaithful to him, that he is being swindled in some outrageous manner, etc., etc. It is characteristic of such delusions, however, that the patient's behaviour is wholly inconsistent with his loudly affirmed beliefs, for though firmly convinced of his wife's adultery, yet he will still continue to cohabit with her.

Irritability and violent outbursts of rage reveal a loss of self-control, and occur most frequently in the bosom of the family, being more or less suppressed before strangers.

In cases of the "progressive dementia" type amnesia is marked from the beginning, the mental faculties fail and the patient becomes dirty and immodest. Hallucinations, mainly aural and visual, are common in such cases, and occasionally delusions may be found, but these tend to disappear as dementia advances.

In the form resembling General Paralysis of the Insane the mental disorders vary greatly. One patient may be in a state of exaltation with markedly grandiose delusions, another depressed and haunted by delusions of persecution, while yet another type may pass into a condition of progressive dementia.

Diagnosis.—The diagnosis between this condition and G. P. I. is at times one of extreme difficulty. A reliable history of the case is of the greatest use to us in solving this problem, as is also the presence of rapidly developed hallucinations and the characteristic physical symptoms, though if physical signs of organic disease be present the question becomes at once a complicated one. A history of syphilis is, of course, an aid, though by no means conclusive for alcoholics, owing to the effects of the drug on their powers of taking care of themselves, are very prone to venereal infection. A differential diagnosis by means of a careful examination of the physical symptoms is our best aid and the main points to be considered are :—

(*a*) *The Condition of the Pupils.*—Inequality and impaired reaction to light may be seen in both conditions, but the presence of the latter is in favour of G. P. I.

(*b*) *Examination of the Fundus.*—Primary optic atrophy favours G. P. I.

(*c*) *Tremors of the Tongue.*—Fine fibrillary tremors favour alcoholism, jerky ataxic movements G. P. I.

(*d*) *Loss of Expression.*—Favours G. P. I.

(*e*) *Speech.*—In G. P. I. is slurred as if the mouth were "full of marbles," and is more hesitating than in alcoholism, where the speech is thick and blurred.

(*f*) *Convulsive Seizures.*—More common in G. P. I.

(*g*) *Knee-jerks.*—Similarly affected in both.

(*h*) *Sensory Affections.*—Much more common in alcoholic conditions resembling G. P. I.

(*i*) *Hallucinations.*—Occur in both, but vivid, visual hallucinations favour alcoholism.

(*j*) *Condition of Tremor.*—Indicative of alcoholism.

Treatment.—The patient must of necessity be deprived of his alcohol, and this is only possible in an asylum or some reliable nursing home, and all attendants on the case must be known to be thoroughly honest and reliable. Some recommend the gradual withdrawal of the alcohol and others its immediate suspension. The latter is, I think, the sounder plan when, as in the majority of cases, the patient's condition permits of it, but where the patients are extremely weak and pulled down such a course is contraindicated, and the alcohol must be withdrawn gradually. Various symptoms arise from the withdrawal which call for treatment. Collapse is by no means infrequent, but forced feeding and drugs, such as caffeine and strychnine, as a rule bring the patient round. Restlessness, nausea and diarrhœa frequently give much trouble and call for the use of sedatives, while insomnia is an invariable and most trying symptom and has to be combated by hypnotics.

All such drugs must however be given with the utmost caution to avoid setting up a drug habit, and I always endeavour to vary the drug as much as possible and avoid letting the patient know what he is getting.

The diet must be liberal, nourishing and easily assimilated and any tendency to refuse food must be at once met by forced feeding.

Prognosis.—Great care must always be taken in prognosticating in a case of this sort, for I have seen most wonderful recoveries when death or complete dementia seemed at one time the only possible termination of the case. Persistent hallucinations are always a bad sign, and in young people marked amnesia is as a rule an unfavourable symptom.

(*e*) Dipsomania.

This, though usually classed among the alcoholic psychoses, is more properly one of the impulsive insanities, such as kleptomania, pyromania, etc., etc. Roughly it may be defined as an impulsive form of insanity, occurring periodically, and manifesting itself in an irresistible craving for alcohol.

In many such cases the patient between the attacks is a respectable useful member of society, often a strict teetotaller, and thoroughly ashamed of his own weakness against which he is constantly striving.

Gradually, however, the craving forces itself upon him, he becomes irritable and depressed, loses his desire for food, and a constant fear of impending trouble casts a shadow over his life. At this time the patient is frantically striving against the craving and frequently implores his friends and relatives to assist him, but, unless such aid is promptly given, the desire proves too strong and a bout of desperate drinking commences. This may continue until an attack of delirium tremens supervenes, though in some cases the drinking may last for a few days or weeks, and then terminate spontaneously for no apparent cause.

A condition of marked depression usually follows after such attacks, during which there is considerable risk of suicide, and this must always be carefully guarded against.

The intervals between attacks vary greatly, sometimes only three or four attacks occurring in a lifetime, but each attack renders a recurrence more probable.

CHAPTER XV.

INSANITIES OF TOXIC ORIGIN—(*contd.*)

Group III.—Insanities due to Drug and Alcoholic Toxines.

INSANITIES DUE TO THE ABUSE OF OPIUM AND MORPHIA.

The consumption of opium is a widespread habit among the inhabitants of India and especially so among the natives of Northern India, but, apart from the misery and want caused by spending hours of every day under the influence of the drug and by the squandering of an enormous amount of money on its purchase, practically no marked mental results accrue, and the number of cases of insanity directly due to its consumption are practically *nil*.

When once the habit has been begun the daily dose is gradually increased, until at last the drug gains such ascendency that its devotee finds it impossible to break from it unaided, and its removal has to be gone about cautiously and with gradually diminished dose to avoid alarming depression and symptoms of heart failure, etc.

In small doses, if its consumers are to be believed, it is often of great use as a restorative after fatigue, a stimulant and a means of obtaining a sensation of general comfort and well-being. Large doses, however, derange digestion, diminish assimilation and so lower the general health, and in this way may undoubtedly prove a secondary cause in the production of insanity.

Apart from this physical result a man addicted to the habit becomes selfish, neglects his duties, wastes his time in the dreamy state caused by the drug which he squanders his substance to procure, is forgetful of his family and of the calls of duty. Beyond this, however, and the intense hold the drug has over him no other mental symptoms occur, and, though treatment in some home or institution is undoubtedly necessary to break him of the habit, his medical attendant would be a foolish rather than a brave man if he were to certify him insane merely for these symptoms. In fact the influence of opium in causing insanity has on the whole been intensely exaggerated, as a glance at asylum statistics in India will convince any one who is inclined to doubt this statement.

Indulgence in Morphia.

Owing to its costliness this is beyond the reach of the average Indian, but among well-to-do Europeans its abuse is fairly common and undoubtedly produces a definite train of symptoms, both mental and physical, for which confinement in an asylum and removal of the drug is undoubtedly the only cure, though at the same time it is an open question whether such cases can be classed as insane or not.

As a rule the habit developes between twenty and thirty-five years of age and both sexes seem equally prone to it. In most cases careful questioning will reveal the fact that the drug was first taken to relieve pain, and the result was found so successful that the operation was repeated on the slightest excuse till the patient found it absolutely essential for his existence. A certain number however there are who have not even this feeble excuse, but take the drug first out of sheer idle curiosity, "just to feel what it is like" as they say, and, finding too late that their power of resistance is weaker than they thought, pay the penalty for their curiosity and become slaves to the drug.

Physical Symptoms.—Prolonged use of the drug produces general gastric derangement with anorexia and constipation. The patient loses weight and becomes sallow and unhealthy in appearance. Salivary secretion is arrested and the mouth becomes dry, creating a feeling of thirst which explains why chronic alcoholism is so often associated with chronic morphinism. The pulse is slow and irregular, and there are frequent attacks of palpitation and threatenings of syncope. Secretions generally are arrested and the skin is dry and loose, but from time to time sudden drenching perspirations seize the patient and render him liable to chills.

Loss of sexual appetite and impotence is present in both sexes when affected by this habit, and in the female amenorrhœa is an invariable concomitant.

Hyperæsthesia is invariably present over the whole body, and in severe cases is so marked that the lightest touch causes the patient to wince or even scream.

The pupils are contracted, their action both to light and accommodation is deficient and defective vision is often present in such cases.

Superficial and deep reflexes are invariably exaggerated, and there is a general lowering of vitality and impairment of muscular power.

Mental Symptoms.—Except for a short interval immediately after the taking of a dose, the general mental condition in such cases is one of depression. Confusion, hallucinations and delusions are by no means common in morphinism where the condition approximates to one of slight dementia with impairment of volition and morality, amnesia and carelessness of personal cleanliness and appearance. Sleep in such cases is most irregular and frequently broken by dreams and visions. Occasionally such cases pass into a delusional condition on which dementia as a rule rapidly supervenes.

If the patient suffers from acute intoxication hallucinations may be present, but these are not often seen unless the drug is combined with cocaine as often happens.

When the drug is suddenly withdrawn a condition closely resembling delirium tremens is caused, the patient becoming anxious and restless, suffering agonies of fear from terrifying hallucinations of sight and hearing, and often passing into a condition of coma and collapse. There is marked anorexia and emesis with abdominal pain and diarrhœa, and often profuse perspiration and salivation. Death may occur in such cases from syncope or collapse.

The feelings of exhaustion and discomfort may persist for weeks after the disappearance of all mental symptoms.

Diagnosis.—This may be by no means easy as morphinists are extremely cunning in concealing their vice. Scars resulting from careless septic injections should be looked for, but the only certain way is to confine the patient to bed in the care of a reliable nurse and wait for the developement of "deprivation symptoms."

Treatment.—This is practically confined to the withdrawal of the drug which may be done suddenly or by degrees. The sudden withdrawal is more likely to be followed by symptoms of syncope and collapse, but in either case the discomfort and misery are the same, only more prolonged by the gradual withdrawal, so one has to make a choice between two evils, and I certainly advocate the former method except when extreme weakness in the patient absolutely contra-indicates it. During the first few weeks of treatment the patient should be confined to bed and fed with milk, eggs, eggflip, meatjuice, &c., and if collapse threatens alcohol, sal volatile or hypodermics of strychnine may be employed. Insomnia, restlessness and discomfort are best allayed by bromides, especially in the form of bromidia. After the disappearance of acute "deprivation symptoms," tonics, cold baths, regular exercise and constant supervision to avoid "backsliding" are required for some months.

Prognosis.—No patients are more troublesome to treat than alcoholics and morphomaniacs, and in no case can one be certain of no relapse occurring. If the patient be in good health and willing to be treated we have a fair prospect of success, but I have known such cases relapse after months of abstinence, so the outlook is never very hopeful.

COCAINISM.

Cocaine is seldom taken alone, but generally combined with morphia to allay the local pain and irritation caused by the injection. Its effects on the nervous system are as a rule more rapid and more marked than those of morphia, but, on the whole, the resemblance between these two conditions is very close, though cocaine poisoning has one symptom peculiar to it, *viz.*, a sensation as of something creeping below the skin, which is especially referred to the fingers and palms of the hands.

Physical Symptoms.—Dyspepsia with constipation and anorexia is invariably present in such cases and general nutrition is much deranged, the weight falling rapidly. The muscles become tremulous and wasted, and occasionally convulsions may occur. Cardiac action is feeble and syncope may threaten to terminate the case. Marked insomnia is invariably present and the patient is continually increasing the dose of the drug to alleviate it. As a rule sexual power is diminished, but occasionally outbursts of eroticism and sexual excitement occur.

Mental Symptoms.—In small doses the drug causes a condition of mild excitement with a sense of increased vigour, in large doses a condition of acute delirium occurs, and with prolonged abuse there is a general failing both of mental and physical power. The patient becomes talkative, suspicious and irritable. His memory and power of attention fail, and vivid hallucinations may suddenly invade his existence without any warning of their approach, and are as a rule of a terrifying, awe-inspiring nature. As time goes on delusions of persecution may develope and the patient resort to carrying lethal weapons to protect himself from his imaginary foes.

Diagnosis.—The sensation of insects or sand under the skin is typical of cocainism.

Treatment.—As for morphinism, but as a rule certification is more often essential here, for the safety of the patients and of others.

Prognosis.—This is fairly good in early cases, but in cases of long standing recovery is by no means common.

ETHER AND CHLOROFORM ABUSE.

The symptoms arising from the abuse of either of these drugs are practically identical with those caused by abuse of alcohol. A single dose of chloroform may in neurotic subjects set up a condition of mild excitement with hallucinations and at times delusions, under the influence of which charges of rape and assault have at times been brought against the anæsthetist.

PARALDEHYDE HABIT.

A knowledge of this is of importance to the alienist as it is one of the most useful hypnotics at his disposal. Its prolonged use as a hypnotic produces a habit so that sleep cannot be obtained without recourse to the drug. It at times produces vivid auditory hallucinations and invariably increases any tendency there may be to hallucinations especially those of hearing.

MERCURIAL AND LEAD POISONING.

Mental symptoms due to chronic poisoning by these metals are practically confined to those constantly working with them and consist of intense mental depression with delusions. At times, however, such cases may be due to badly kalaied cooking pots, as the kalai is sometimes applied mixed with lead.

The classical physical symptoms of chronic poisoning, such as salivation, a blue line round the gums, peripheral neuritis, constipation and diarrhœa, neuralgic pains, headache, paresis and muscular tremors should be well known to all medical men and need not be gone into fully here. In the same way there is but little need to discuss the treatment of such cases which are practically unknown in India except for the few which may arise from badly supervised cooking utensils.

IODOFORM POISONING.

This is at times met with as the result of surgical dressings, etc. The condition is one of low muttering delirium with tremors of the voluntary muscles and lasts for about three weeks, recovery as a rule being perfect.

CARBON-BISULPHIDE POISONING.

Occurs commonly among those working with rubber. The physical symptoms are those of marked malnutrition and anæmia, while mentally the condition is one of delusional insanity with at times vivid auditory hallucinations. The treatment is mainly tonic, iron and arsenic being especially serviceable in such conditions. Recovery generally ensues, but the condition tends to be chronic, and as a rule has a long course, lasting for over a year. Relapses are sure to occur if such cases return to their former work after recovery.

THYROID POISONING.

This results as a rule from the prolonged administration of thyroid extract in nervous cases. The condition is generally one of transient excitement without confusion and soon passes off when the drug is discontinued.

CHAPTER XVI.

NERVOUS DISORDERS COMPLICATED BY MENTAL DERANGEMENTS.

EPILEPSY.

This is a condition of the utmost importance to a medical man, not only from a medical, but also from a medico-legal point of view.

Epilepsy has been defined by Gowers as "a nervous disease characterised by a sudden discharge of nervous energy from the grey matter of the cerebral cortex, this discharge occurring without normal stimulus."

To understand this condition fully a knowledge of the microscopic structure of the motor area of the cerebral cortex is necessary, and as the disease is a common one in India among all classes of the community, and an important one, too, for the medical practitioner, I will venture to describe its origin as briefly as possible.

Histologically the cerebral cortex is generally described as consisting of five layers of nerve cells.

1. A superficial layer with abundance of neuroglia and a few small multipolar nerve cells.
2. A thin layer of a large number of closely packed small nerve cells of pyramidal shape.
3. A very thin layer of numerous large pyramidal cells, each with a process running from the apex vertically towards the free surface and lateral processes

at the base which are always branched. There is also a median process from the base of each cell which is continuous with a nerve fibre. The bundles of fibres spread out in this layer.

4. Numerous nerve cells, some large and some small, forming a layer known as Meynert's "granular formation."

5. Spindle shaped and branched nerve cells of moderate size, arranged as a rule parallel to the free surface. This layer is broken up by fibres passing in groups to the outer layers.

The developement of these cells and layers differs markedly in the various cortical regions. In the sensori-motor area around the fissure of Rolando, which is the area with which we are at present concerned, the large pyramidal cells of the third layer attain their maximum developement and large cells are plentiful in the fourth layer. The pyramidal cells of the third layer are those from which the motor or efferent fibres originate.

Under normal conditions the large pyramidal cells of the third layer are, according to Bevan Lewis, constantly producing energy which is kept under control by the small pyramidal cells of the second layer until some approximate stimulus causes the release of a proportionate amount of energy from the cells of the third layer, either by its direct action on these cells or indirectly through the cells of the second layer having their controlling action inhibited for the time being. Holding this view Bevan Lewis, who has made a careful study of the brains of epileptics, states that he believes epilepsy is due primarily to change in the cells of the second layer whose nuclei first show changes of a fatty nature, the whole cell finally undergoing vacuolation and as a result becoming unable to control the energy produced by the cells of the third layer which is, as a result, discharged spasmodically producing the fits so well known to all medical men. This is, however, but pure theory so far as I know, and, as Bevan Lewis himself admits, such a condition is not peculiar to epilepsy, and most authorities now look on it as of either immediately *ante mortem* or *post mortem* developement.

The latest theory on the subject and one with a good deal to support it is the theory of the toxic origin of epilepsy. The grounds in support of this are varied. Thus the temperature of epileptic patients is irregular and liable to become febrile at intervals, independently of any outward bodily or mental symptoms. The pulse is also liable to similar irregularities affecting its rate, its rhythm and its tension. The leucocytosis and results of blood examinations before, after, and during the fits, also strongly favours this toxic theory of its origin, thus the polymorphonuclear percentage falls and there is a corresponding eosinophilia immediately before the appearance of a fit, after which the polymorphonuclear percentage rises above normal causing a temporary hyperleucocytosis. These changes in the blood point more to an auto-intoxication from deranged metabolism than to a bacterial toxæmia. Moreover several European scientists have recorded that the urine drawn from epileptic patients during a fit produces convulsions when introduced into the venous circulation of animals.

As to the nature of the toxine, this is still a matter of conjecture. Haig regards it as due to uric acid poisoning, and it is an undoubted fact that the uric acid excretion falls before a fit and that a corresponding rise occurs in the excretion after the fit is over. Krainsky however holds the view that the essential irritant is carbonate of ammonia and brings forward strong evidence to support his theory.

Whatever may be the nature of the essential irritant, however, it is certain that in epileptics metabolism tends to be imperfect ; the average excretion of azotised products, phosphoric acid and chlorides is below normal in the interconvulsive periods, and is still further diminished in the prodromal periods.

After a fit the urine is more concentrated, contains a larger proportion of all the regressive products of metabolism and is much more toxic than normal urine when injected into the lower animals. In the period immediately preceding a fit this toxicity of the urine increases greatly and is proportionate to the amount of gastro-intestinal disturbance present, while after a fit the urine is hypertoxic. Gastro-intestinal disturbances seem to favour the formation of the toxine and indeed seem able to determine the occurrence of a fit, as the use of gastric lavage, intestinal disinfectants, purgatives, etc., etc., is a great aid in holding the fits in abeyance.

The gastro-intestinal changes consist chiefly in the occurrence of abnormal putrefaction among the contents of the alimentary tract, and the amount of this occurring can be roughly obtained by an estimation of the amount of ethereal sulphates excreted in the urine, which invariably increases prior to the occurrence of a fit.

Along with the accumulation of toxines in the blood there is in such cases a corresponding diminution in the alkalinity of the blood.

How these toxines act, whether directly on the nerve cells themselves, or indirectly by producing cerebral congestion or anæmia by vasomotor spasm, is still unknown, but it is, I think, universally admitted now that there are two undoubted factors in the production of epilepsy :—(*a*) a special defect of cerebral organisation which predisposes to the epileptic discharge, (*b*) a toxic action which determines this discharge.

Ætiology.—Hereditary predisposition to nervous diseases is very marked in these cases, being present in well over 50% of patients. Age, too, has a considerable influence on the appearance of this disease, more than 75% of cases occurring in the first twenty years of life, of which about 35—40 per cent. occur in the first decennium. The sexes are affected practically in equal proportions.

The exciting causes are various. It may arise from a bad brain habit following the occurrence of infantile convulsions, cerebral injuries or sudden mental shocks may suffice to originate it, as also mental anxiety and strain, while at times it occurs as a sequel to such acute specific diseases as scarlet fever.

Symptoms.—Physical. The physical health always suffers much in cases of epilepsy. There is, as a rule, gastric derangement, evidenced by furred tongue and constipation, nutrition is impaired and loss of weight ensues, while sleep is restless and broken. Automatism is a common condition in epileptics, especially in the Petit Mal, and, as a rule, follows the fit, the patient invariably going through the same movement or action immediately after the seizure while still in a condition of unconsciousness.

The fits are the most important physical symptoms and may be described as of three types: 1. *Grand Mal*, or major epilepsy, where the fit is of severe character. 2. *Petit Mal*, where the fit is comparatively mild in character. 3. *Jacksonian Epilepsy*, where the convulsions affect primarily one limb and spread from thence to the whole body.

1. *Grand Mal.*—Here occasionally there is an aura or warning, the patient having hemicrania, various neuralgic pains, gastric discomfort, localised analgesias or some other sensory manifestation immediately prior to the fit. As a rule, however, the fit comes on suddenly, the patient, with a cry, due to the forcible expulsion of air through the glottis, falls helplessly to the ground in a state of tonic convulsions. The tonic convulsions after 20—30 seconds pass into the clonic convulsions, in which the muscles move in violent jerks, the tongue is apt to be extruded and bitten, and the patient foams or froths at the mouth. The condition of clonic convulsions passes into one of more or less marked stupor with stertorous breathing which passes into normal sleep from which the patient awakes with no recollection of anything which occurred during the seizure. As a rule such patients on awakening are

confused and dull and complain of muscular pain and stiffness.

2. *Petit Mal.*—In its typical form this consists of a temporary loss of consciousness, without visible convulsions or spasms, during which the patient may or may not fall to the ground. On returning to consciousness the patient may at once continue his occupation as if nothing had happened, or may be confused and ask what has happened or what he was doing. These minor seizures are very apt to recur and several may ensue in the course of a single day. The tendency here too is for the mental faculties to fail rapidly, and if definite mental disorder supervenes the physical health as a rule becomes speedily impaired.

3. *Jacksonian Epilepsy.*—This condition was first described by Hughlings Jackson, from whom its name was derived. In it the muscular spasm commences locally in a hand, finger or foot, and may be localised to this one region. As a rule, however, the spasm tends to spread until the whole body is involved and insensibility supervenes, though at first, when the spasm is localised, there is no loss of consciousness.

Status Epilepticus is a term applied to very severe forms of the *Grand Mal* where the seizures occur in rapid sequence, consciousness does not return in the intervals between the fits and a fatal termination is very frequent.

Mental Symptoms.—Many epileptics go through life without showing symptoms of mental derangement beyond being at times unduly irritable, impulsive, passionate and emotional, especially on religious questions. When, however, mental disease does supervene it is practically always excitement with more or less marked confusion. The predisposing cause in such cases is undoubtedly the inherent or acquired mental deficiency which allows the occurrence of the sudden discharges of nervous energy which constitute the epileptic spasms, while alcoholic excesses, mental shock and strain figure as the chief exciting causes. Once an epileptic has suffered from even the most transitory mental derangement there is always a liability of its recurrence, and each attack increases this tendency and favours the occurrence of the same mental symptoms over and over again.

The earlier mental derangements are generally short bouts of acute excitement from which the patient as a rule completely recovers, but gradually as the attacks continue the mental equilibrium becomes more and more impaired until a condition of chronic mental derangement is attained, characterised by hallucinations and delusions, wild excitement, loss of self-control and obsessions and impulses which are usually homicidal, though occasionally they may be suicidal in character. Such cases are very liable to perverted religious emotionalism, and when in their religious moods are more liable to outbursts of frenzied rage and virulent abuse than at other times.

The moral sense is blunted in most epileptics and such cases are invariably most untruthful and vindictive.

Sexual desire is commonly intense in such cases and gives rise to masturbation and brutal assaults and outrages. Many of these patients are gluttonous and given to over-eating and alcoholic excesses.

In most cases of long standing there is always more or less mental enfeeblement which may pass into dementia of a most degraded type.

Insanity associated with Epilepsy.—Various types of insanity may be associated with epilepsy.

1. *Epileptic Idiocy or Imbecility.*—This may arise from arrested mental developement caused by convulsions in early life.

2. *Pre-epileptic Insanity.*—Occurs in certain cases where the mental symptoms precede the motor convulsions.

3. *Epilepsie Larvée (Masked Epilepsy).*—In this condition the motor convulsions are replaced by the mental disturbance, an attack of insanity taking the place of a fit, though some authorities state that a fit invariably occurs but is so slight that it is overlooked in these cases.

4. *Post Epileptic Insanity.*—This occurs as a sequel to the motor convulsions and is generally of a very severe type.

5. *Chronic Epileptic Insanity.*—This is the most common form of insanity met with in epileptic patients.

In addition to the above mental conditions epileptics are liable to suffer from other acute insanities just as are other individuals, indeed with the epileptic the liability is rather greater on account of the marked hereditary taint present in so many persons thus affected, and also from the deranged metabolism weakening the natural resistance of the healthy body to bacterial invasion and laying the patient more open to suffer from toxæmias.

1. *Epileptic Imbecility and Idiocy.*—These cases arise from the mental developement having been retarded by the occurrence of epileptic fits in early childhood, and dentition is as a rule the exciting cause in such cases.

Such patients are usually very impulsive and irritable and require careful supervision to prevent their injuring children with whom they may associate. If the fits continue long there is generally marked mental deterioration, but the fits may continue for some years without causing any marked intellectual degeneration, and if treatment be successful in arresting the fits there is in most cases marked improvement in the mental condition.

2. *Pre-epileptic Insanity.*—This is practically a mental aura replacing the sensory ones which have been mentioned in the description of the *Grand Mal.* Hallucinations of sight and hearing terrify the patient and give rise to delusions, under the influence of which assaults may be perpetrated and false charges formulated against entirely innocent persons. There is generally considerable excitement present in this condition and refusal of food is frequently met with in such cases. The mental attack may precede a fit by a few hours or a few days.

3. *Masked Epilepsy.*—This is a term used to denote cases where there are no apparent convulsions, the fit apparently being replaced by mental symptoms. Cases of automatism have been classed by some under

this head, but now it is generally admitted that the automatism is, as a rule, preceded by a slight fit.

4. *Post Epileptic Psychoses.*—These are of various kinds and are of the utmost importance to the medical jurist, on account of the frequency with which acts of homicide have been committed by persons suffering from this condition. In such cases the stupor which usually follows after the fits may be replaced by a period of automatism. Such patients are, as a rule, confused, fail to recognise their nearest relatives and wander aimlessly about, openly committing crimes of nearly every kind, and in such conditions brutal homicides and sexual assaults are very common, the patient on recovery rarely remembering anything he may have done.

In such cases of crime there is in most instances no traceable motive, and no attempt at concealment is made at the time of perpetration, though later, with returning consciousness, fear may give rise to efforts at concealment. There is moreover an unnecessary violence and brutality about such crimes, by which I mean a much greater amount of force and violence is shown than is necessary for their perpetration. This should at once give rise in a medical mind to a suspicion of the true state of affairs, and a careful enquiry into the antecedents of the culprit will generally bring forward ample corroborative evidence.

In some cases a violent attack of mania replaces the coma, and while in this condition the patient is in a state of frenzy, shouting, kicking, biting, scratching and committing even homicidal assaults on any and every one.

As a rule this condition is quite transitory lasting for a few hours only.

In a still smaller number of cases a period of mental depression follows after the fits. In such a condition delusions of persecution are common and may lead to acts of homicide or suicide.

5. *Chronic Epileptic Insanity.*—The general tendency of epilepsy is towards a gradually progressive dementia. Memory fails, self-control is diminished, outbursts of passion and anger, exaltation and excitement alternate with periods of misery and gloom. The patient becomes arrogant and boastful, and, though full of religious professions and always forcing religion upon others, their whole character, their every action belie their sermons. Morals are conspicuous by their absence in such patients, liars, drunkards, and men given to the lowest forms of vice and sexual excesses, comprising the most degraded type of case to be seen in any asylum.

Diagnosis.—The diagnosis of epilepsy is by no means invariably an easy matter, especially when the fits are of the *Petit Mal* type. The seizures, too, often occur at night and the history in such cases may be very obscure. Careful enquiry should be made for unconscious micturition or defæcation, and the tongue examined for scars and signs of injury, in such patients. Sudden erratic conduct, incompatible with the former character of the patient, should always suggest epilepsy to the medical mind, and cause a closer supervision to be kept on the patient. Hysteria and epilepsy are at times difficult to distinguish in the earlier age periods, but the former almost invariably occurs when the patient is in company and is commonly set up by some external influence, while the fall is not so helpless nor so liable to result in injury as is the case in epileptic fits. In place of the subsequent stuporose condition also there is in hysteria a condition of extreme emotionalism and grotesque attitudinising which never occurs in epilepsy.

In later life a diagnosis has to be made between true epilepsy and the congestive seizures so common among general paralytics. In such a case the state of the pupils, the speech, the handwriting, reflexes, etc., must all be carefully gone into and a careful enquiry made regarding the onset of the seizure, as in G. P. I. the onset is as a rule more gradual and the epileptic cry is wanting.

Treatment.—Much depends on the general hygiene of the patient's surroundings in cases of epilepsy. The diet should be simple, fattening and non-stimulating, and over-feeding must be carefully avoided. Alcohol, flesh, tea, coffee and tobacco should be given only sparingly or, better still, withheld altogether. The bowels should be carefully regulated and saline purges administered at intervals, while the patient should be encouraged to drink water freely so as to flush out noxious substances from the system. Regular open air exercise should be insisted on whenever practicable, the patient's life should be kept as quiet and as routine as possible, and all undue excitement avoided.

Medicinally the only drugs of any service are the bromides, the bromide of potassium giving perhaps the best results. They are usually given in 30 grain doses thrice daily after food and should be continued for long periods without a break.

Richet and Tolouse introduced recently an ingenious modification of the bromide treatment, based upon the theory that the privation of chlorides intensified the absorption of similar salts by the body cells. They therefore reduced the amount of chlorides in the food as far as possible, placing their patients at the same time on about 50 grains of sodium bromide daily with the result that the fits in these cases were largely reduced while under the treatment. I myself have tried withdrawing sodium chloride from the diet of such cases and replacing it with potassium bromide, and the result is most satisfactory, though unfortunately I have not enough statistics to quote from. In my cases moreover, except for the removal of the chloride, the diet is the same as that issued to the rest of the native patients and must contain a fair amount of chlorides in itself. Only 10 grs. of pot. brom. is issued for each epileptic twice daily. This reduces the number of fits to a practically negligible number, the patients improve both physically and mentally, and bromism is unknown.

Bromism is apt to be troublesome after a lengthy course of the usual treatment, acute eruptions, gastric disturbances and lethargy troubling the patient. In such cases purgatives and hot baths are indicated, while liquor arsenicalis 2—5 mins. or salol 2—5 grs. combined with the bromide tends to avert the trouble. In severe cases soda biborate 2—10 grs. thrice daily combined with liquor arsenicalis 3 mins. is most effective.

Other sedatives, such as nephente, belladonna, Indian hemp, nitroglycerine and erythrol tetranitrate are all useful at times, especially in cases of *petit mal* in young persons.

When a sensory aura occurs in a limb the subsequent fit can often be wholly arrested by tying a ligature tightly round the limb.

In cases of status epilepticus chloroform inhalations are worth trying, also inhalations of nitroglycerine or erythrol tetranitrate, or hypodermic or rectal injections of chloral hydrate, but very rarely is any benefit derived in this condition, death generally occurring from hypostatic congestion of the lungs.

Epileptic cases always require careful supervision to prevent injuries occurring in the fits, to avert choking if the fit occurs during a meal or to avoid suffocation arising from the patient, during a state of stupor, turning over with his face on a pillow, etc.

Mental symptoms may at times be aborted by 5 grs. of calomel followed by a saline purge, or 1 min. of croton oil, if the excitement is coming on gradually, or the patient is given to over-eating and only has occasional attacks. Where mental symptoms follow after a fit 20 grs. of chloral combined with 30 grs. of potassium bromide may produce sleep and thus cut short the mental attack.

Prognosis.—Major epilepsy or *Grand Mal* is a much more curable disorder than the *Petit Mal*, and if it developes in childhood may often be successfully treated, though as the treatment is often a question of years it is difficult at times to get the patients to continue with it. Epilepsy resulting from gross brain lesions and also *Petit Mal* are practically incurable.

CHAPTER XVII.

NERVOUS DISORDERS COMPLICATED BY MENTAL DERANGEMENTS.

General Paralysis of the Insane (*G. P. I.*).

This condition is occasionally seen among Europeans and Eurasians in India, though it is said to be very rare among natives. I purposely use the qualified term here, for though in the *Indian Medical Gazette* for January 1912 this disease is said to be very rare among natives, and though I can find no record of any such having been admitted into the Agra Asylum in previous years except in very old records, yet during the hot weather 1909 I had two patients admitted, one from Dehra Dun, a *gharrami* by caste, and the other a Mussalman from Jhansi, both of whom seemed to me typical cases of this condition. One of these cases died about January 1910, after I had returned to my regiment. A *post mortem* was done and the condition said to be due to a hæmorrhage into the internal capsule. No microscopic examination of the brain was made, however, nor was it attempted to find the cause of the hæmorrhage, so I consider my diagnosis by no means disproved.

The second case died in January 1911, and I was fortunate enough to be present at the *post mortem*. No marked coarse lesions of the brain or meninges were present, but sections were sent home to Dr. Ford Robertson with a full statement of the case, and from his report there is absolutely no doubt of the correctness of my diagnosis in this case, and the probability of the first case also being correctly diagnosed is to my mind strengthened by this report. At present there are 3 typical cases of this disease, in the second and third stages, in the Agra Asylum, and since November 1911 one case has died in a typical congestive seizure, and another, in the early stages, has been taken out by his friends. So that I am of the opinion that if properly looked for and diagnosed it would be found to be much more prevalent among natives than it is at present generally believed to be.

The disease may be defined as a progressive degeneration of the central nervous system, but more particularly of the motor centres, in which remissions and arrest of progress of the symptoms are common, epileptiform or convulsive seizures often occur, and with which there is always associated a progressive mental enfeeblement.

G. P. I. is almost invariably fatal, the patient dying during a congestive seizure, from some intercurrent disease such as phthisis or pneumonia, or as the result of exhaustion from advanced paralysis or bedsores.

Patients suffering from this disease are liable to attacks of any known form of insanity; indeed, according to Dr. Bruce, it is only very rarely that cases uncomplicated by mental disease are met with. This cannot be too strongly impressed upon the mind, for so frequently is it complicated by mental symptoms that many alienists have jumped at a wrong conclusion and described as one entity what is really two separate conditions, classing G. P. I. among mental diseases, when, from their description, they are really dealing with two diseases, a purely nervous one and G. P. I. complicated by an intercurrent attack of some form of insanity.

Ætiology.—General Paralysis is seen much more frequently among urban than rural populations and affects men more often than it does women. It may occur in childhood, adult life or old age, but is most commonly and typically seen in men from 35—45 years of age. Only a small number of cases (7—8 per cent.) have a hereditary nervous taint, but from 70—90 per cent. have a history of acquired syphilis, and all the cases I have seen which occurred in the age periods up to twenty have either had a history of congenital syphilis or, if this was denied, had all the physical stigmata of this condition.

The theory of an auto-intoxication of syphilitic or para-syphilitic origin was at one time strongly combated by Ford Robertson and others who promulgated the theory that this disease, and also locomotor ataxy, were due to the toxines produced by a diphtheroid bacillus, which they described as of 2 types: (*a*) the B. paralyticans longus; and (*b*) the B. paralyticans brevis. This latter theory had at one time a fair number of adherents, and if it be well-founded undoubtedly opens up a new field in the treatment of mental disease. The opinion at present generally held however is, I think, that the proof regarding B. paralyticans and its action is insufficient, and the tendency to regard G. P. I. and locomotor ataxy as terminal syphilitic manifestations is present in the majority of medical authorities.

Symptoms.—For purposes of description this disease is best divided into four stages—(*a*) Prodromal ; (*b*) First Stage ; (*c*) Second Stage ; (*d*) Third Stage. It must be remembered, however, that there is no fixed line of demarcation, the disease being gradually progressive and the one stage merging unnoticeably into the other.

(*a*) *Prodromal*—**Physical Symptoms.**—Before the definite onset of general paralysis there are as a rule certain more or less definite symptoms lasting for some months or even years. The patient changes in habits and character, becomes either restless and unusually energetic, or torpid and sluggish. Alcoholic and sexual excesses are common at this stage and are often wrongly interpreted as causal factors instead of symptoms. Definite complaints of gastric derangement, neuralgic pains, numbness and transient changes in hearing, vision, taste and smell are often made, while passing attacks of aphasia, paresis affecting the muscles of the eyes, causing strabisums and diplopia, or of the extremities are very suggestive of this condition. Attacks of syncope and congestive seizures, often mistaken for epilepsy, may occur early in this disease.

Mental Symptoms.—The mental symptoms at this stage are not marked and might perhaps escape the notice of a total stranger. There is a general impairment of the more specialized powers of the brain, a loss of memory and of the power of attention, associated with a lack of judgment and a failure of volition which renders the patient liable to be led astray, to fall a prey to any swindler and to plunge into absurd and foolish speculation. A loss of self-control leads to violent outbursts of rage and undue emotionalism, while honesty and morality are at a low ebb and the patient is liable to commit thefts and other more criminal offences.

Occasionally G. P. I. may begin suddenly with marked mental or motor symptoms. The mental symptoms may be either of an excited or of a melancholic type, while the motor may present the form either of an epileptic seizure or of some form of paresis. In whatever way the condition first manifests itself, however, physical symptoms soon reveal themselves and the diagnosis is apparent.

G. P. I. being, as already stated, more a nervous than a mental condition, it is proposed to discuss the physical symptoms of the three remaining stages first and consider the mental symptoms thereafter.

Physical Symptoms :—(*b*) *First Stage.*—In this period of the disease the facial muscles are commonly affected causing an alteration in expression, while the evening temperature runs from 99°—101°F., falling to normal in the morning.

At times there are marked symptoms of gastric derangement, constipation being often a source of great trouble, but in other cases the patient enjoys comparative freedom from these and eats well. The pulse is rapid and irregular, the arterial tension high, while the leucocytosis, as already mentioned, is irregular with, as a rule, a high polymorphonuclear percentage. There is an exaltation of the sexual instincts in the earlier part of this stage, but later on these may be in abeyance. Sensibility to touch and temperature and also the special senses are rarely affected in this stage, but in about 50% of cases sensibility to pain is diminished. The condition of the pupils varies greatly. As a rule the pupils are unequal in size and irregular in outline, varying in size and shape from day to day. In some cases reaction both to light and accommodation are lost, in others the Argyll Robertson pupil may be present. The pupils may be contracted to pinpoints or widely dilated. One pupil only may show signs of being affected while the other may appear normal. In fact no definite condition of the pupil can be laid down as characteristic of this condition for any and every condition of pupil may occur. The superficial reflexes are exaggerated as are also the tendon reflexes, except in cases with marked tabetic symptoms or those complicated by chronic alcoholism. There is general impairment of muscular movement throughout the whole body, causing marked inco-ordination and affecting more especially the muscles of the face, tongue, hands and lower limbs. The paresis of the facial and tongue muscles leads to loss of expression and a typical slow monotonous speech with slurring of the labials, or if the lingual muscles are more affected there is a blurred murmur as if the patient had his mouth full of marbles, such phrases as "dusra lumba rissala," "apka bap ka nam," being pronounced with difficulty. The muscular impairment of the hands and arms causes loss of co-ordination and of the finer movements, such as writing, etc. The gait is sometimes dragging, sometimes ataxic, but the patient always has difficulty in walking along a straight line, in placing one foot in front of the other, or in turning quickly, lurching or swaying occurring when any of these are attempted. Many patients too are unable to stand with their feet together and with closed eyes, and very few indeed can rise on tiptoe with their eyes shut.

During this stage the patient loses weight and insomnia is apt to be troublesome.

(c) *Second Stage.*—Here the involvement of the facial muscles is still more advanced, the face being absolutely expressionless, no matter what the mood of the patient may be, and at times being pallid and puffy as in cases of kidney disease.

The temperature chart, in complicated cases, shows every second or third week recurrent attacks of slight fever, and gastric derangements are practically the rule. Appetite is often enormous and at times perverted, the breath is exceedingly offensive, the tongue coated and furred, and alternating attacks of constipation and diarrhœa may prove an endless source of worry to the patient. The leucocytosis corresponds fairly well to the curve of the temperature chart, the polymorphonuclear percentage however as a rule remains about normal, the main increase, when the leucocytosis rises, being in the eosinophiles and the hyalines, so far as my experience goes.

The pulse is slow with a high arterial tension and attacks of syncope are liable to occur especially after a heavy meal or during exercise. The skin is unhealthy, greasy and œdematous, and the hair and nails rough and brittle. Diminished sexual instinct and impotence are common in this stage and form a marked contrast therefore to the first stage. Sensation, both general and special, is now much involved. The muscles are much more markedly affected and paretic, tremors are very apparent and inco-ordination, etc., are well marked throughout the body. Congestive seizures are common throughout this stage, and are liable at times to be mistaken for epileptic seizures. Their incidence corresponds closely to the febrile attacks. During this stage the patient very commonly puts on weight, but the gain is not a healthy one, the tissues being loose and flabby. Primary optic atrophy is very common in such cases, and at times commencing symptoms may be found in the first stage even.

(*d*) *Third stage.*—The claim of G. P. I. to be classed as a progressive nervous disease is undoubtedly most marked in this stage, emaciation and loss of power advancing with amazing rapidity. The face is thin, wasted and expressionless, gastric derangements are practically the rule, diarrhœa and vomiting being constant and most troublesome factors to deal with. The temperature during this stage is most irregular, at times rising in the evening to 99°—100°F., but as a rule being subnormal. The pulse is extremely feeble and irregular, arterial tension is low and cyanosis and œdema of the extremities is common and the lungs are apt to become tubercular. During this stage the leucocytosis is most irregular and shows no association with the temperature, the polymorph percentage however is as a rule low, below 50 per cent., while the hyalines and eosinophiles always figure high in the count. The skin has the unhealthy look of old parchment and trophic changes are manifest in the appearance of boils, carbuncles and bedsores. Common sensibility is practically lost and the special senses are all more or less affected. Paralysis is now marked and the patient is practically bedridden. Urine and fæces are voided unconsciously, and it is with the greatest difficulty the patient can be kept clean, while constant supervision may have to be exercised to prevent his choking over food owing to impairment of the reflex act of swallowing. In the end of this stage the patient is a helpless, useless lump of what one can scarcely call humanity, and the disease soon terminates either from a congestive seizure, pneumonia, accidents or exhaustion.

Mental Symptoms.—In uncomplicated cases of G. P. I. the characteristic mental condition is one of gradually progressive enfeeblement terminating sooner or later in dementia. As a rule however there is such marked derangement present that it is commonly believed that G. P. I. is invariably associated with insanity, or is in itself a type of insanity. Almost every type of insanity has at one time or another been described as associated with G. P. I., but in the majority of cases these mental symptoms have been intercurrent with and not symptomatic of the nervous condition.

The mental symptoms recognised as typical of the disease however are elevation with grandiose delusions.

In the first stage the patient seems endowed with superabundant energy and an overpowering sense of well-being and self-satisfaction. There is slight mental confusion, and impairment of judgment leads to the wildest statements and delusions, and to the patient's launching out into the wildest projects and speculations; consciousness and the power of cognition remain however practically unimpaired. Loss of self-control leads to undue irritability and emotionalism, and when combined, as is generally the case, with an impairment of the moral sense, may be the cause of theft and other criminal offences. Memory is untrustworthy and the power of attention is impaired leading to incapacity for occupation. Such patients are, as a rule, garrulous but not incoherent, and the false sense of well-being leads to voluminous writing of poetry or imaginary business letters. Hallucinations are rarely, if ever, present in uncomplicated cases. Sleep occurs at times naturally, but in most cases this function is deranged, while nightmares are common in the earlier stages of this condition, which on the whole corresponds fairly well to the simple elevation of folie circulaire.

As the physical symptoms of the *second stage* become manifest the mental symptoms alter. *Pari passu* with the advancing paresis there is marked mental enfeeblement, the patient is less energetic and restless, and the general intelligence is markedly impaired. The special senses are less acute and there is therefore less response to external stimuli; delusions, however, similar to those in the first stage, may persist, but they are as a rule less prominent and do not affect the conduct so markedly. The tendency to theft is increased, but the efforts of the patient are misdirected and large piles of rubbish are accumulated which could be of no use to anybody.

The patient becomes listless, careless of his appearance and easily managed, while the advancing paresis and mental enfeeblement put an end to the volubility and the incessant writing of the first stage.

The mental symptoms of the second pass gradually into those of the *third stage*. The patient becomes more and more demented, gradually losing all human instincts and interests in life until he is practically a mass of flesh, only kept alive by the constant care and attention of others. Congestive seizures are extremely common and as a rule hasten the mental decay, though in one or two cases I have seen a distinct improvement in the mental condition occur after such an attack.

Diagnosis.—This is by no means always an easy question to decide. The conditions most likely to cause us trouble are chronic alcoholism, cerebellar tumors, epilepsy, disseminated sclerosis and poisoning by lead, chloral or cocaine. In such questionable cases the only thing to do is to place the patient under careful observation, for some months perhaps if necessary, note carefully his behaviour and physical and mental condition from time to time and also the results of treatment.

Treatment.—Certain European and American alienists are experimenting with the diphtheroid bacillus already noted, and two at least claim to have produced a serum which has most beneficial results. Further and more convincing proof however is required before these, or even the B. paralyticans, can be accepted by the faculty generally.

Meanwhile such cases are treated on general hygienic principles and attention is mainly directed to combating the symptoms and alleviating pain and distress. The question of home-treatment is often raised in connection with this disease, and though possible in some cases, I cannot say I ever approve of it, especially in the early stages, for such patients are, at first at least, capable of begetting offspring, and it is most undesirable, both for the possible progeny and the general public, that this should occur. I therefore strongly recommend asylum treatment in all cases in the early stages of the disease, or, where the patient can afford it, removal to some quiet place, in the hills if possible, where he can have good attendants to care for him and will be away from his family as much as possible. In the later stages, quiet demented cases can be quite suitably treated at home, but restless excitable patients are much better in an asylum.

The diet should be stimulating and fattening and alcohol should be entirely withdrawn. Tobacco may be allowed in the earlier stages, but should be withheld as the disease progresses as it is then very liable to cause nausea and syncope. Constipation should be constantly looked for and laxatives given where occasion arises. Restlessness and excitement, if acute, call for the use of sedatives and sulphonal grs. x, pot. brom. grs. xxx morning and evening are the ones I have found most serviceable in such cases. Sleeplessness should be treated with hot baths, hot draughts of milk at bedtime, hot bottles applied to the feet, etc., before hypnotics are resorted to, as these often suffice to give a quiet restful night, and by their means we can avoid having recourse to drugs.

Antisyphilitic treatment is rarely of benefit in such cases, but it should invariably be given a trial. Personally I have no experience of the Salvarsan injection in such cases, but in the Medico-Psychological Journal for January 1912, I see that Salvarsan, though extremely useful in early syphilitic nervous manifestations, is worse than useless in cases where there is any sign of dementia as it merely seems to hasten the mental decay. Hence its use seems contraindicated in G. P. I., but liq. hydrarg. perchlor. m. xl and pot. iod. grs. v to grs. x is my favourite prescription in such a condition.

Prognosis.—The duration of G. P. I. is extremely variable, one case may die within two months of the onset of the acute symptoms, while others may hang on for 10 or even 20 years. As a rule however three to four years may be looked on as the average duration of a case. Much however depends on the character and cause of the remissions; thus if a remission be due to an acute intercurrent disease, such as pneumonia or erysipelas, it may be of long duration and lengthen the course of the disease by months or even years. Recovery from this condition is at present unheard of.

CHAPTER XVIII.

STATES OF MENTAL ENFEEBLEMENT.

1. Idiocy and Imbecility. 2. Dementia.

States of Mental Enfeeblement may be due either to arrested developement or to structural changes occurring in the grey matter of the cerebral cortex.

If the condition be due to failure in developement or structural changes in early life it is termed *Idiocy or Imbecility*, whereas if it result from acute brain disease, gross brain lesions or old age, it is known as *Dementia*, and classified into *secondary dementia*, *organic dementia* or *senile dementia* according to the cause.

1. IDIOCY AND IMBECILITY.

Ireland defines these conditions as follows:—"Idiocy is a mental deficiency or extreme stupidity, depending upon malnutrition or disease of the nervous centres, occurring either before birth or before the evolution of the mental faculties in childhood. Imbecility is generally used to denote a less decided degree of mental incapacity."

Ætiology.—The ætiology of these two conditions can be treated of under two heads: (1) Pre-natal, (2) Post-natal.

1. *Pre-natal Causes.*—A *neurotic inheritance* exists in a very large percentage of such cases, insanity, epilepsy,

alcoholism and syphilis being commonly present in one or both parents.

Phthisis or other wasting diseases in the parents may be the determining factors of idiocy in the progeny. Syphilis, if contracted by the parents several years before the birth of the child, is not so liable to cause imbecility, but if the father be suffering from syphilis at the time of the conception or the mother during her pregnancy, then the outlook is much more serious.

The influence of *alcoholism* as an ætiological factor here has given rise to much controversy, but, on considering the number of children who though not actual imbeciles still show more or less marked stigmata of degeneracy, one can but conclude that alcoholism is undoubtedly potential as a factor in the production of this disease, both directly as well as indirectly, by lowering the natural resistance of the organism and rendering it more liable to be affected by other causes.

Consanguinity has often been brought forward as a strong factor in the production of this condition, the laity especially being convinced of this. As a matter of fact consanguinity only acts by emphasizing and exaggerating weak points in the mental and physical characters of the parents, any failing common to both parents being more pronounced in the offspring and more liable to be handed down through succeeding generations.

The *age of the parents* has an undoubted effect, however, for not only are the offspring of very youthful and very aged parents liable to show signs of physical and mental deterioration, but the offspring of parents of unsuitable ages, where a large series of years intervene between husband and wife, or *vice versâ*, are also liable to be similarly affected.

During gestation any severe shock or accident, especially if the woman be of a neurotic type, may suffice to affect the fœtus in utero and produce an idiot, and a similar result may occur if the mother, during pregnancy, contract any acute specific disease.

Prolonged labour causing protracted pressure on the cranium is an undoubted cause of imbecility, especially among first-born children, and accounts in a measure for the predominance of male over female idiots, as male infants are commonly larger than female. *Injuries by instruments* during parturition are similarly responsible for a certain percentage of cases.

2. *Post-Natal causes.—Infantile convulsions,* no matter how they originate, are responsible for a very large number of cases of weakmindedness, not only from the damage and deterioration they produce in the nervous tissues, but also as they tend to arrest further developement and the child subsequently remains mentally enfeebled.

Gross diseases and traumata of the brain and meninges are responsible undoubtedly for a small number of such cases, while the influence of the *acute specific fevers* as scarlet fever, whooping cough, diphtheria, etc., is still more marked and widespread.

Lastly in some cases imbecility may be largely due to *careless upbringing* and *bad home influences and education.*

Thus the conditions likely to cause imbecility and idiocy are numerous and varied, and, as a rule, it is impossible to say that any one factor alone is responsible for this state as two or three are generally acting in combination and forming as it were a "vicious circle."

To sum up the matter, therefore, we may say generally that, *imbecility is due to anything which arrests cerebral developement and the evolution of the complex nervous elements and the associated fibres which connect these centres with one another.*

Cause and effect must be carefully distinguished when we consider such conditions, thus at one time in microcephalic idiots the cause was considered to be a premature ossification of the cranial sutures, whereas now observation has shown us that the primary condition is a failure in the cerebral developement which allows the premature ossification to occur.

Symptoms.—Various classifications of idiocy and imbecility have from time to time been promulgated, thus Ireland classifies the condition into various types according to the ætiological factors causing the arrest of developement, whilst others classify them according to the severity of the symptoms and the extent to which mental developement has proceeded. In the former the difference is mainly ætiological and in the latter merely one of degree, and there is practically no difference between the symptoms of any two types, so that I propose firstly to consider the symptoms broadly and as one class. In doing so I would warn my readers that various grades of intensity in the symptoms are met with every day, from the idiot whose mind is practically a blank and who is incapable of learning, to the individual who though simple-minded has yet acquired some elements of education and may even be an adept at carving or some other mechanical occupation. Having done this then a few lines will suffice to complete the various ætiological and other types.

Physical Symptoms.—The physical symptoms of idiocy and imbecility are mainly what are known as *stigmata of degeneration* and include abnormalities and deformities in practically every region of the body. The stature is frequently below the average in size and the long bones unduly curved. The skull may be unduly large, or abnormally small and misshapen, or symmetrical. Thus the forehead may be receding and give a pointed appearance to the head, or a non-developement of the occipital region may cause the cranium to appear flattened. Premature ossification of the sutures may occur from arrested cerebral developement, or the converse may occur as in hydrocephalic cases.

The palate is, as a rule, high, narrow and V-shaped, and a receding lower jaw is such a common concomitant that even the laity on seeing a man with such a feature are apt to exclaim "What an idiot he looks."

The teeth are generally badly formed, and readily decay, while they are frequently crowded together and rarely show the complete complement.

The orbits may be either too close together or too widely apart, and at times approximate to the Mongolian type, while the pupils may be oval in shape. Strabismus and other visual defects are common.

The ears may be abnormally situated, or the pinna badly formed, or the rim, the helix and other ridges and fossæ in the cartilage deformed or wanting altogether.

Congenital valvular deficiency is very common in the hearts of such cases, while, as a rule, the circulation is feeble and the fingers and toes cyanosed.

The tonsils are frequently hypertrophied in such cases and adenoids are extremely common. Food is generally bolted without proper mastication and causes dyspepsia. Constipation due to altered or deficient intestinal secretion is often seen, but at times obstinate diarrhœa may prove a source of endless worry. Hence nutrition in these cases is usually bad and, in conjunction with the shallow respiration so common in the imbecile, renders them specially prone to phthisis and other pulmonary troubles.

The skin is often coarse and the subcutaneous tissues thickened. The hair is thin and brittle, frequently absent from the faces of male idiots, but often present to an excessive extent on the faces of females. Pubic hair is commonly scanty or absent in both sexes. The nails are brittle and badly formed.

Various malformations of the genital organs are met with in such cases, and in females menstruation occurs very late or may be entirely absent. Sexual instinct is at times in abeyance, but more frequently it is abnormally strong and leads to masturbation and other vicious practices.

Sensation is dulled, and from this and sluggish mentalisation the superficial and organic reflexes are affected, saliva dribbling from the mouth, owing to the impairment of the pharyngeal reflex, while the acts of micturition and defæcation are absolutely uncontrolled, and such patients are as a rule very dirty.

Motor phenomena are numerous and interesting. In infancy the microkinetic or spontaneous uncontrolled movements seen in healthy babes are absent, and the child is either abnormally quiet and motionless or else goes through more automatic regular movements than the spontaneous ones performed in health. The voluntary movements are slow and badly performed, co-ordination is generally markedly deficient and such children are very late in learning to walk, while more marked cases never learn to dress themselves. Muscular debility and paralysis of every kind is very common in these cases, and may render standing or walking impossible, while tremors may be present, either localised to one or other extremity or implicating the whole body.

Speech is markedly impaired in all cases of any intensity, and even in the milder forms is invariably very late in developing. This impairment is due in the vast majority of cases to defective cerebration, though in a certain number it is undoubtedly due to defects in the respiratory or laryngeal mechanism, and, as a rule, these latter cases are much more easily instructed and managed. Stammering is common among imbeciles, but deafmutes are little if any more numerous than they are among the general population.

The features are, as a rule, coarse, out of proportion, and the head misshapen, while the expression in the majority is most degraded. Many are continually grimacing and laughing, others again look sullen and morose, while a vacant, senseless expression is found in some cases. Attitudes and postures are invariably awkward and clumsy, while the gait is waddling and the whole personality devoid of grace.

Many of such cases seem to be in a condition of continual torpor and drowsiness, spending practically the whole of their time in sleepy inactivity, in others, however, the converse is to be seen, a condition of restless activity prevailing, and the hours passed in sleep being few. Dreams and night-terrors are very common among imbecile children.

Mental Symptoms.—The power of memory varies greatly in idiocy and imbecility, but even in the most intellectual of such cases there is invariably seen deficiency in this faculty. The causes of this are manifold; thus as a rule such patients have a difficulty in associating ideas, and memory largely depends upon this. Lack of the power of concentrating the attention, too, is common among such cases and has an undoubted effect on the memory, but probably the lack of language and "word ideas" is chiefly responsible for this condition in the majority of imbeciles. In some of the feeble-minded however a highly specialised memory is present, which is, however, practically useless as it seems to be developed at the expense of all other faculties.

Attention is one of the faculties of later developement in the healthy child, and in the weak-minded mental developement is usually arrested before this faculty is fully acquired. Even passive or spontaneous attention, the first and most primeval form, on which we rely as a safeguard against sudden dangers, may be absent in some idiots and, as a result, their powers of self-preservation are at a minimum. Inattention may be due either to defective cerebration, or to defective sense organs or their afferent fibres interfering with the strength of the stimuli which reach the brain. In some cases the stimulation of one sense organ may not suffice to attract the attention, but if the stimuli are such that they can act on two or more of the senses at once then attention is attracted, and this is specially the case when the visual sense is one of those acted upon.

Deficiency or perversion of one or all of the special senses is one of the common characteristics of idiots, and not only accounts for the difficulty experienced in training such individuals, but also is very largely responsible for the failure of mental developement, as it is by sensation that knowledge is first acquired.

Idiots are as a class wholly devoid of emotion or sentiment, and it is only in the highest types of such cases that any great depth of feeling is developed. The idiot in fact responds merely to physical and not to moral pain, and, as a rule, is incapable of cherishing any feeling for a long time, the enemy of to-day being the friend of to-morrow and *vice versâ*; I know, however, of one or two cases where the reverse has been the case and extraordinary love or hatred has been shown by the patient for some particular person, and with absolutely unselfish motives too.

Religious feeling is absent in practically all idiots whose thoughts are wrapped up in the present with no comprehension of a future. Morals too are markedly deficient in such persons, they lie and steal openly and apparently without knowing they are doing wrong, and are, as a rule, most inquisitive, while many have an overweening idea of their importance which renders them easy dupes of unprincipled persons. A few of the higher imbeciles are extremely vain and dress outrageously and extravagantly, but, as a class, the tendency is to marked carelessness of the personal appearance and clothing. The lower instincts, being free from central inhibitory control, run riot and lead to gross dissipations and brutal cruelty at times to children and animals, and many idiots are extremely passionate and reckless, though others again are very docile, and, learning what pleases those in charge of them, always endeavour to please them.

The behaviour and conduct of the weak-minded varies greatly. In the lowest types we meet with helpless individuals unable to feed or clothe themselves, who can take no interest in anything, can do nothing, and are dependent on those around them for their very existence. From this lowest level there are varying grades, shading impalpably into each other, from those unable to attend to the lowest functions of the body, to those whose sole defect seems an inability to acquire knowledge of the social and moral laws of the community.

As regards the capacity for occupation and earning a livelihood, this, as can be readily imagined, is most variable. The lowest class of idiot is quite unteachable, and in fact seems at times to delight in destroying things, sometimes from sheer love of destruction, at other times aimlessly and more for the sake of distraction and to pass the time. Next to these come those who are late in acquiring knowledge and are incapable of any but the simplest occupation, but are yet able to maintain existence in their own particular line. In the higher types we meet with the "one-sided genius," the "wonderful infant musician," the "mathematical wonder," etc., etc., which are all of this type, the one talent seeming to be developed at the expense of all other mental powers.

The great difficulty in teaching imbeciles is their inability to concentrate their attention, but once a trade or craft is learnt they generally prove excellent workmen, as they pursue their calling in an automatic sort of way and are not easily led away from it.

The judgment, owing to lack of the power of observation, want of memory, deficient powers of attention and absence of emotionalism, is deficient in all imbeciles to a greater or less extent.

Types of Idiocy.—The types of idiocy usually described are: 1. *Genetous.* 2. *Mongolian.* 3. *Microcephalic.* 4. *Hydrocephalic.* 5. *Hypertrophic.* 6. *Eclampsic.* 7. *Epileptic.* 8. *Paralytic.* 9. *Traumatic.* 10. *Inflammatory* or *post-febrile.* 11. *Syphilitic.* 12. *Cretinoid.* 13. *Idiocy from deprivation of the senses.* In India practically all these types are recognisable, and I have met with examples of them all, except the cretinoid, but even it is seen at times, though apparently less commonly than in Europe, as Major Ewens, I.M.S., notes in his book on Insanity that it occasionally is met with in India. Another class, however, requires mention in Indian psychiatry, and that is the individuals already described (Chapter VIII) as "Shah Daula's Mice," for, though corresponding closely perhaps to the microcephalic type, yet there are certain differences which set them apart as a separate type and a distinct entity in themselves.

1. *Genetous Idiocy.*—Is the term applied by Ireland to congenital idiots, for whose mental deficiency no cause, beyond perhaps hereditary defect, can be assigned. Deformities of head and limbs are by no means common in this class though many are stunted in growth. The child, as a rule, has a dull, degraded expression, the ears are large and defective, the palate is high and narrow and the teeth bad, while the gait is clumsy and ungraceful. Rickets and scrofula are frequent concomitants of this condition. In many of these cases, if the circulation and nourishment be good, sensibility not markedly impaired, and the power of attention present, there is a fair hope of educating the child to a certain extent and training him to some simple trade or occupation.

2. *Mongolian Idiocy.*—This is practically a subdivision of genetous idiocy and draws its name from the physiognomy of such cases and the great resemblance they bear to the Chinese. The head is small and rounded, the features broad and the eyes placed slantingly in the face. The figure is dwarfed and stunted and the hands and feet broad and clumsy. Organic disease of the heart is very common among such cases and the circulation in all is feeble. Such individuals are usually good-tempered and imitative, but have very little intellect, and there is practically no hope of training them to any trade or occupation, however simple it may be.

3. *Microcephalic Idiocy.*—In these cases the head is always unduly small, and it may be taken as an axiom that where the cranial circumference is less than seventeen inches it is a sure indication of idiocy, though the condition is due more to arrested brain developement than to cranial malformation. In this class of case the head is narrow and oxycephalic in shape, and the subjects are usually unduly active and restless, though strange to say they are, as a rule, late in learning to walk. The large majority are very quarrelsome and aggressive and are very deficient in mental capability and in the power of attention, so that it is practically impossible to educate them to even the simplest occupation. Morals and the sense of propriety are usually conspicuous by their absence in such cases.

4. *Hydrocephalic Idiocy.*—This must be distinguished carefully from the hypertrophic variety with which it is very liable to be confused, but the shape of the head differs in certain particulars and enables one to make certain of the diagnosis. It must be always remembered, however, that a large head does not always connote hydrocephalus and that many normal children have abnormally large heads. I know indeed of a case where a father, who was himself a medical man, for some months underwent all the horror of believing his only child a hydrocephalic imbecile, and the grandfather too, also a medical man, when he saw the child on his arrival in England, experienced a similar shock. The condition was fortunately wholly different, and the child has developed into a bright intelligent boy without a single moral or intellectual taint.

As a rule the hydrocephalic head is rounded in shape, the widest diameter, if any, being situated about the temples, and the fontanelles are raised, whereas in rickets the anteroposterior diameter is the longest and the fontanelles are depressed. Hydrocephalus may cause death in early infancy, a few cases recover, but in the large majority the child hangs on a hopeless idiot and usually blind or deaf or both from the intracranial pressure. Such cases are generally good-tempered and friendly, and a certain number may be educated to a slight extent, but the prognosis is practically hopeless as regards teaching them an occupation.

5. *Hypertrophic Idiocy.*—This is due to an abnormal development of the white matter of the cerebrum. The head is, as a rule, square, or elongated anteroposteriorly, the greatest width being above the superciliary ridges. The head never attains the size of a hydrocephalic head. The condition is very rare in India and usually developes in early life. Individuals affected thus suffer from frequent headaches, are slow in their movements and cannot learn readily. They can, however, be educated to a certain point, and many in time are capable of supporting themselves by some simple occupation.

6. *Eclampsic Idiocy.*—Here the condition is due to infantile convulsions, arising from teething or some other stress. Such cases are usually excitable and passionate, and, though they may seem bright and intelligent enough, owing to their abnormal restlessness and lack of power in concentrating the attention, it is practically impossible to educate them. The progno-

sis depends largely on the extent and severity of the convulsions, and where these have been fairly mild some small hope may be given to the parents. Such cases are, as a rule, devoid of morals, and their sense of propriety is at an extremely low ebb.

7. *Epileptic Idiocy.*—Epilepsy invariably tends to produce weak-mindedness, either in early life by arresting evolution, or in later life by causing a process of dissolution. The fits may appear at any age, but in the majority of cases of epileptic idiocy they occur about the time of teething. Shuttleworth and Fletcher Beach divide such cases into three classes: (*a*) Bright well-made children, who progress at school and take an interest in their work, whether educational or industrial. (*b*) Children who are also well-informed, but are listless, though they can talk and take an interest in what is going on around them. These cases, as a rule, progress well for a time and then a succession of fits comes on and they become dazed and stupid losing much of of what they have already learnt. (*c*) Cases which, on account of the frequency of fits, make little or no progress with their education.

The faces of such children are commonly dull and more animal in type, and they approximate to the lower grades of idiocy. Such cases, as a rule, are passionate and violently impulsive, and require careful supervision to prevent their harming their playmates. They form by far the largest class of imbeciles in Indian asylums, and though the prognosis varies somewhat with the frequency and intensity of the seizures, it is never by any means hopeful.

8. *Paralytic Idiocy.*—In this type of case the damage to the brain may be either pre-natal or post-natal. The paralysis is, as a rule, one-sided and the arms are generally more affected than the legs, the muscles being in a condition of spastic rigidity. I have, however, seen cases, indeed one is at present under my care, where both arms and legs are affected and the patient is absolutely helpless. In the majority of such patients there is great impairment of the mental faculties and education is impossible, but in a certain number of the milder cases a small amount of education may be possible.

9. *Traumatic Idiocy.*—This form may be due to protracted labour in a woman with an abnormally small pelvis, to injury caused by instruments during labour, or to a blow or fall on the head after birth. The degree of mental incapacity is proportional, as a rule, to the amount of damage done to the brain, but at times an apparently slight injury may be followed by very severe symptoms. Cases where the injury occurs during birth are usually the most pronounced and incapable of being educated, while those in whom the injury occurs after birth may be physically strong, and even learn how to read and write, but retain the mind of a child throughout their whole life and are only fit for the simplest occupations.

10. *Inflammatory Idiocy.*—This occurs as a sequel to the acute specific fevers which are liable to set up inflammation of the brain and its membranes. The amount of mental deficiency is directly proportional to the amount of damage done to the cerebral tissues and many cases improve greatly under careful training.

Where, however, much damage has been done to the brain the child remains degraded, irritable and uncontrollable and cannot be taught.

11. *Syphilitic Idiocy.*—Hereditary syphilis is by no means a common cause of idiocy. As a rule the mental symptoms develope late, the child at first merely showing the physical symptoms common to such a condition and otherwise developing normally until about 8 or 10 years of age, when convulsive seizures supervene, mental developement is arrested and a definite deterioration ensues.

12. *Cretinoid Idiocy.*—This type of idiocy is occasionally met with in the hills and villages where goitre and other affections of the thyroid gland are common. The infant appears at first normal, but as developement proceeds physical abnormalities and mental deficiencies become apparent. Growth is retarded as a rule and the figure becomes squat and dwarfish with short thick limbs and slow clumsy movements. The skin is dry and harsh, the eyelids swollen and the lips and tongue thickened. Dentition is delayed and the teeth are badly placed and readily decay. The voice is harsh, and speech slow and limited as regards the vocabulary. The abdomen is flabby and protuberant from changes in the subcutaneous tissues, and the sexual organs as a rule are small and ill-developed. The circulation is feeble and such cases constantly complain of being cold. These patients are usually good-tempered and affectionate, but their mental capacity is of the poorest and they can be taught only by the exercise of much perseverance and patience.

Under thyroid preparations a marked improvement occurs in most cases, but the patient must continue the treatment throughout his life or he will relapse into his former condition. During the administration of the thyroid preparations careful supervision must be exercised as in some cases rapid loss of weight ensues, while in others the temperature rises rapidly, there is great increase of the pulse rate, and severe diarrhœa may terminate in a collapse.

13. *Idiocy from deprivation of the senses.*—To produce this condition an absence of two at least of the more important senses, such as sight and hearing, is essential. It is always possible to teach such children, and in Britain, where there are special institutions for such sufferers, remarkably good results are obtained. In India, however, without such institutions and few, if any, people with the proper training and knowledge for educating such patients, the task is practically a hopeless one and the prognosis in such cases is very far from hopeful.

14. *Shah Daula's Mice.*—This is a type of idiocy peculiar to a certain district in the Punjab and has already been described (*vide* Part I, Chap. VIII).

Treatment.—The treatment of idiocy covers a wide field, as it includes not only the treatment of the various factors which may have caused the arrest of developement, but also the physical, mental and moral training of the patient.

All possible causes of this condition must be carefully looked for and steps taken for their proper care and treatment. Nutrition is of the utmost importance in all such cases, and having arranged for the treatment of the cause, our care must next be directed to the diet. The food should be simple and largely farinaceous, meat being avoided as much as possible. Many idiots are given to overeating and bolting their food in masses without properly masticating it, and such cases must have their meals supervised by a nurse or some responsible person to prevent choking, or the gastric derangements which will otherwise inevitably occur. The clothing of such cases is also a matter requiring attention, for many are acutely sensitive to cold. It should be light but warm therefore and, in cases given to masturbation or exposing their persons, garments like pyjamas, made without any opening in front and of stout material, are often most useful.

In many cases the teaching of cleanliness is a most difficult matter, and it may be months before the child gives any sign when he wants to attend to the calls of nature. In older cases bathing in cold water, or withdrawing some luxury, whenever he offends thus, has often a wonderful effect in stimulating the memory. Personal ablutions and dressing are also matters requiring instruction. The former is best done by carrying out the ablutions at regular fixed times, some one being always at hand to see that the cleaning is properly performed; dressing however is a much more difficult performance and quite beyond the powers of many idiots.

Swedish drill, etc., are of great use in developing the patient both physically and mentally, but such exercises should always be carefully regulated and supervised so as to avoid unduly fatiguing the patient.

Mental training must in these cases be begun gradually, and our first aim should be to develope the acuteness of the various senses as far as possible and to strengthen the power of attention. Sight can be developed by using coloured balls and boxes and making him put the balls into similarly coloured boxes, or matching coloured bricks or wools, etc. Hearing can be rendered more acute by means of musical notes, bells, etc. Touch is a sense requiring careful attention, it should be begun in the first place by coarse movements such as putting ninepins or balls into sockets, etc., then smoothness and roughness can be explained by velvet and a file, and similarly sharp and blunt, hot and cold things can be explained to him. A most important lesson and one that cannot be taught too early is that fire burns, and proper care given to expounding this may avert serious accidents in later life. Finer movements may be taught as the child progresses by making him string small beads or do a little simple careful work. The senses of taste and smell are less important, but should be developed by means of various scents and solutions.

Attention is at times most difficult to attract, and much trouble is at times necessary before the child seems to gain the slightest control over it. Our efforts should invariably be directed to this object at first, for until some power is acquired in this direction practically nothing can be done. Brightly coloured or glistening articles, loud sounds, heat and cold, and failing these even mild electrical shocks, may all be resorted to that we may achieve this object.

Learning to walk is always a difficult task for the weak-minded and the difficulty is due to various causes. In some the capacity to understand or to imitate may be wanting, while in others the incapacity may be due to some nervous or muscular defect. Thus it is a matter of importance to ascertain in each case where the deficiency lies. Many and varied are the mechanisms evolved for the purpose of teaching such cases to walk, the most useful of which are especially constructed swings, or circular supports on wheels. Where muscular weakness is one of the obstacles to be overcome massage is an invaluable aid in the treatment.

Learning to speak is a great difficulty in all such patients, and generally they can understand what is said to them long before they seem to acquire the power of expressing themselves, probably because of a lack of ideas and thoughts to express. In all such cases the respiratory apparatus should be carefully tested and all defects, such as adenoids and enlarged tonsils, rectified and removed as far as possible. Thereafter the child should be put through regular breathing exercises and carefully trained to distinguish sounds. Thereafter the labial and lingual movements should be shown to the patient who should be made to imitate them from the teacher. In this way the child gradually extends his vocabulary, advancing by degrees from monosyllables to words of two or three syllables, until he can pronounce a complete sentence and express himself fairly clearly. The extent of the vocabulary that can be learned varies, however, greatly in the different types of idiocy, and, as a rule, it can be accepted as an axiom that if a child does not learn to speak before the age of six or seven, his vocabulary will always be of the smallest.

Writing is a much more difficult accomplishment than speaking on account of its greater complexity, and is far beyond the powers of the majority of idiots. Copying or even tracing of lines or figures is the best means available, but it must be remembered that an idiot may be able to write a word or even a series of words purely mechanically and without the slightest comprehension of the significance of his action.

Industrial education is a matter of the utmost importance in the raising of such individuals, and it is in this respect that we are so lamentably handicapped in India by a complete absence of special asylums for the poorer patients of this class, and of kindergartens for those higher in the social scale and able to pay for their training. Many of these children have a wonderful aptitude for some special work, such as carving, and yet are wholly unfit for any other occupation however simple. As a rule, however, farming or agriculture is the work for which such persons are best suited, and with careful supervision most excellent results may be obtained in this line.

Moral training is perhaps the most difficult though at the same time the most important, and no one who is not endowed with unlimited patience should attempt the post of teacher to an imbecile. Such children are abnormally apprehensive and timorous, and one's sole hope of success is by gaining their affection, for by this alone have we any hold over them, corporal punishment being, in the majority of cases, not only useless but actually harmful. Good behaviour should be rewarded from time to time with little luxuries or rewards, and misconduct similarly rewarded by a withdrawal of these, but punishment should go no further. A thing to be remembered too in such cases is the lack of the sense of morality which is practically invariably present, and careful supervision must always be exercised in order to avert some possibly serious catastrophe.

Many such cases are full of professions and promises, and mean them too at the time, but barely are the words uttered than they are forgotten, and the child is quite likely to transgress again quite innocently in the presence of his teacher.

One can thus readily imagine what an uphill task the training of such a child is, and how much patience and perseverance is required to tackle it. Through it all however one has the knowledge that even the most hopeless cases may eventually learn something, and if this can be accomplished the greatest reward one can have is to hear the child talking, perhaps calling to one in terms of affection, and to realise that part at least of the dark shadow has by one's efforts been removed from the little sufferer.

DEMENTIA.

Dementia or secondary dementia is used, in contradistinction to primary dementia, amentia or idiocy, to denote a condition of weak-mindedness due, not to arrested developement, but to progressive deterioration resulting either from gross brain disease or from degeneration of the nervous elements of the brain. A former state of higher intellectual power is therefore denoted by the term and, provided life lasts long enough, it may be looked on as the final mental condition of us all.

The word "dementia" has been applied by various authors to many conditions with a complete disregard of the possible duration of such conditions and whether they were permanent or merely temporary in character. Such a use of the word is not only unscientific but most confusing, and it is really more accurate and simpler in every way to look upon it as a distinct and separate entity, not as a disease in itself, but as merely the last and permanent mental state towards which so many of the acute insanities tend. Dementia is best classed under two heads :—1. *Secondary Dementia*. 2. *Organic Dementia*.

Secondary Dementia may be described as a state of mental enfeeblement, which may ensue after an attack of any of the acute insanities, and which has certain definite symptoms of its own, though these may be affected to a certain extent by the persistence of some of the characteristic features of the original mental disorder. The depth of mental enfeeblement may vary widely, from mere inattention and loss of the power of concentrated thought to a condition of profound degradation.

Ætiology.—A neurotic heredity is usually traceable in all such cases, and they are usually found most typically after those types of insanity which are most prone to occur in early adult life, and in which a neurotic heredity is a common, if not a constant factor. Alcoholism and epilepsy are especially liable to terminate thus.

Symptoms.—As a rule, when an acute attack of insanity is passing into dementia, there is a marked improvement in the physical condition without any similar change in the mental symptoms, and when this condition occurs one should never be led astray and give rise to false hopes in the minds of the relatives, who are only too apt to be misled by it themselves. It should be explained to them carefully and tactfully that the mental prognosis is now even less hopeful than before the physical improvement, and they should gradually be brought to an understanding of the true state of affairs. As the condition advances appetite and sleep improve and often the weight increases enormously, though if excitement and restlessness persist both the powers of nutrition and sleep remain deranged. Some dements, however, remain in a continual state of ill-health. Their circulation is feeble and their extremities cyanosed and cold. In some the appetite is voracious, but nutrition is deranged and weight is in consequence lost rather than gained, whilst in others a degraded appetite leads to the eating of mud, sticks, leaves, stones and every kind of rubbish. The features of such cases are coarse and degraded, and the gait slow, clumsy and shambling. All finer co-ordination is lost, and movements are in consequence slow and clumsy.

In short, the patient is mentally and physically degenerate; he looks degraded, his thoughts and actions are of a lower type than formerly, his appetites are perverted, his sensations dulled and his lower instincts, being no longer under control, run riot, and what may have formerly been an intelligent, useful member of society becomes a moral and intellectual wreck and a heavy charge upon his relatives or the State.

Mental.—The mental symptoms of dementia vary greatly in intensity. In all such cases there is diminished self-control and the patients are usually irritable and easily aroused, but a little tact quickly appeases their rage and restores them to good humour again. Such patients are very apt to lose their powers of cognition and of adapting themselves to circumstances, and thus are at a loss to support themselves in life, though in an institution, such as an asylum where life is regular and work properly supervised, such a man may prove most useful, working automatically almost day after day, apparently quite happy in his occupation and never thinking of asking for a holiday. Advanced cases are, however, practically unfit for working, and if they do find anything to keep them busy, it is as a rule in the destructive rather than the constructive line.

The feelings and emotions are always affected in cases of dementia, subject-consciousness and object-consciousness both being diminished, and provided such cases are comfortable for the time being they have no thought of anything else, the deaths of friends and relatives bring forth not the slightest sign of grief, they may even be threatened with hanging next day, and the only result is a grin or a demand for some little luxury. At times such cases may be most importunate in their demands to be sent home, but such a phase is but momentary and a passing butterfly or the stub of a cigarette is quite sufficient to drive the idea out of their heads and for months one may never hear of it again. In cases, the sequel to acute attacks of mania, maniacal outbursts may occasionally occur, while others again have an air of arrogance and decorate themselves most fantastically.

Where the mental enfeeblement is at all marked, the conversation and actions are as a rule most degraded, and to this type belong those wretched individuals so common in Indian Asylums and commonly spoken of as "mud-eaters." The cause of this condition—mud-eating—is still under investigation, and various theories are promulgated at present, such as a deficiency of calcium chloride in the system, or a deficiency of iron, with the result that a craving is induced for material from which such salts can be derived. I have enquired carefully into the matter and have heard on good authority that round about Moradabad about 5 per cent. of the villagers are addicted to this habit, "eating mud as if it were a sweetmeat," and my informant also stated that though such men did not look markedly unhealthy prior to acquiring the habit, they soon fell off in health, and in a few years were wretchedly weak, anæmic individuals and fit for nothing, and as ankylostoma duodenale is found here present in practically all such cases of *post-mortem* it is small wonder such is the case. A similar condition is sometimes to be noted in pregnant women, and I have known cases where European ladies during pregnancy clamoured for chalk and eat it greedily, and here I think the theory of a deficiency of calcium chloride is quite tenable. Among "mud-eaters" in asylums, however, I am strongly inclined to think the condition simply due to depraved appetites, for if put into pucca barracks and removed from all chance of obtaining earth they simply take to eating anything they can get hold of, sticks, leaves, cloth, paper, everything being crammed into their mouths. Many of such cases are terribly anæmic, I have seen cases where the percentage of hæmoglobin has fallen as low as 12 per cent., but when placed under proper supervision, and given good nourishing food, iron tonics, the phosphates and at times calcium chloride, the improvement in physical health is marked. So soon, however, as the supervision is relaxed, no matter how fit the patient may be, even with cent. per cent. hæmoglobin, no matter if the tonic, etc., be still continued, he relapses into his former habits, and in a year or so, if left to his own devices, is back to the same debilitated state.

The memory is always affected in dements, but in some cases, though recent memory be practically *nil*, the memory for past events may be extraordinary, minute details which occurred over twenty years before being most accurately stored in their minds.

Dements, owing to their extreme facility and liability to be duped by unprincipled persons, are as a rule incapable of looking after their affairs, but many are quite fit to make a reasonable will and one that will be recognised by law, and this must always be borne in mind and great care taken when one is called in for such an object.

Homicidal and suicidal acts may occur from time to time in such cases, especially the former, and, as a rule, are due to sudden impulses, the patient being incapable of elaborating any definite plan of attack, or indeed of cherishing any ill-will for any length of time.

Treatment.—With careful supervision and hygienic surroundings marked improvement may occur in many of these cases. It must be remembered that the minds of such persons approximate closely to that of a child and much may be done to *educate* them, not only to cleanliness, and a sense of morality and common decency, but even to some useful occupation. Thus at the present moment most of the gardening, etc., of asylums is done by dements who are supervised by the warder staff.

(*b*) **Organic Dementia.**—This is the term applied to mental enfeeblement arising from some gross lesion of the brain. The lesion may be diffuse or localised, and the intensity of the mental symptoms is due as much to the site of the lesion as to its extent. Mental symptoms are one of the many concomitants of such conditions and are fairly late in developing, being as a rule preceded by various motor manifestations.

Where the lesions are diffuse, as in chronic meningo-encephalitis, a progressive mental deterioration is the rule with marked loss of memory and derangements of speech. Such patients are generally irritable and liable to outbursts of violent maniacal excitement, while convulsive seizures may occur. The pulse in such cases is rapid and irregular, and arterial tension low, and many of these patients die from syncope or exhaustion.

Where the lesion is localised, as in cerebral tumours, hæmorrhages, embolisms, abcesses, etc., the later stages of the condition are always marked by more or less pronounced mental changes, and at times mental symptoms may be an early and important manifestation of the disease. In chronic cases, where the tumour growth is slow, the most common condition is one of gradually increasing lethargy and somnolence. Such cases think and speak slowly and with difficulty, their movements are slow and awkward, they take no interest in their surroundings and have apparently no interest in life, and certainly seldom seem to have any wants or desires.

In cases of acute onset, as in hæmorrhage or embolism, where sudden alteration in the intracranial pressure occurs, the mental symptoms are much more acute. Restlessness and delirium are common in such conditions, and hallucinations of sight and hearing often terrify the patient. Lesions of the frontal lobes are more liable to be accompanied by early mental symptoms than are lesions in other parts of the brain, but it must be remembered that a growth may exist in the frontal lobes and yet give rise to no mental derangement whatsoever. Localisation, though at times possible from motor manifestations, is practically impossible from mental symptoms alone. The rate of growth of the lesion is of importance as regards the mental symptoms, a rapidly growing tumour giving rise to more numerous and more marked mental disturbances than one of slow growth.

In by far the majority of such cases a careful enquiry is sure to elicit a history of neurotic heredity.

Physical Symptoms.—The physical symptoms depend mainly on the character and site of the lesion and will be found in any text-book on medicine, so need not be described here.

Mental Symptoms.—Progressive loss of memory and of the power of cognition are the most common mental concomitants of organic lesions of the brain, and may render the patient totally unable to look after himself and apparently regardless of common decency. As the disease progresses the mental condition increases more and more, and the patient finally becomes bedridden and hopelessly demented. In cases of cerebral hæmorrhage I have at times seen severe emotional disturbances, both of excitement and depression, and in one case it seemed the starting point of a series of maniacal attacks, and the patient is now in a state of comparative dementia with periodic exacerbations of excitement.

Diagnosis.—This can only be made from the physical symptoms and is often a matter of difficulty. At times the mental disturbances are the first symptoms noticed and may lead to the patients being sent to an asylum without the true condition having been diagnosed. Hysteria and G. P. I. may at times be confused with such states.

Treatment.—Syphilitic cases and those where operative interference is practicable are the only patients where treatment is possible, and for the rest careful supervision and nursing with general hygienic treatment is all that can be done.

Prognosis.—Except in syphilitic cases or where operation is possible the prognosis is hopeless, and even in these cases the outlook is by no means favourable.

CHAPTER XIX.

PSYCHOSES ASSOCIATED WITH PHYSICAL DISEASES.

Psychoses associated with Physical Diseases are as a rule classifiable under the head of Exhaustive Insanity, Insanity due to Metabolic Toxæmia, Insanity due to Bacterial Toxæmia or a combination of these, and I am doubtful as to whether such a chapter as I propose this to be is, strictly speaking, scientifically accurate. It is an undoubted fact however that many physical diseases have certain mental characteristics or concomitants, a knowledge of which is most useful to the physician, not only from a psychiatrical point of view, but also as it affects his treatment of and bearing towards the patient quite apart from any question of sanity or insanity. For this reason therefore I propose in this chapter to describe the mental conditions found in some of the common physical diseases and run the risk of being dubbed scientifically inaccurate.

I. Phthisis and Insanity.

Apart altogether from insanity there is a peculiar mental attitude associated with cases of phthisis; no matter how ill the patient may be he is always full of hope as to his ultimate recovery, and this hope I have known to persist in cases practically till death. This being such a prominent feature in such patients who are mentally sound, it might be supposed that in cases where insanity was a sequel to the physical condition the mental state would be one of excitement, exaltation or elevation. Such however is not the case for, as a rule, such patients suffer from a mild depression with delusions of persecution and suspicion.

In considering such cases it must always be kept in mind that though phthisis is such a common cause of death in asylums in by far the majority of such cases the physical disease is secondary to the mental one and may even have been contracted after the patient's admission, and has nothing whatever to do with the mental condition. It is only when insanity is consecutive to the lung disease that this state of delusional depression is seen, which is however by no means pathognomonic of phthisis.

The relationship between phthisis and insanity is a close one, a tubercular parent begetting children, some of whom are tubercular, while others may be insane, while tuberculosis finds a much larger percentage of victims in asylums than in the general population.

Mental Symptoms.—Where the insanity is consecutive to the physical disease, the patients as a rule are peevish and irritable, and many are depressed and unable to settle to any occupation. Delusions are common and may lead to refusal of food so that tube-feeding becomes necessary. The power of self-control is diminished and the power of attention and concentrated thought is lost, though memory is little if at all impaired and if so mainly for current events.

Attempts at suicide are common in such cases and have to be guarded against.

As the case progresses a condition of partial dementia ensues, but often when the pulmonary trouble is far advanced and life is nearly at an end there is a sudden and marked improvement in the mental condition which may continue until the moment of death.

Diagnosis.—The diagnosis of phthisis in an insane person is a matter of no little difficulty as a rule owing to the difficulties experienced in auscultation. Generally rapid loss of weight, especially if accompanied by an irregular febrile chart, should make us suspect this condition.

Treatment.—Beyond careful supervision and artificial feeding, if necessary, nothing beyond the ordinary treatment for phthisical patients is called for. I always endeavour to keep such patients away from non-tubercular cases, and so far as possible have the expectoration collected and destroyed. They should be kept as much as possible in the open air, under a shelter, and a plentiful supply of good nourishing food allowed to them.

Prognosis.—This depends largely on the extent of the lung trouble, but is generally by no means hopeful.

II.—Malaria and Insanity.

As with other specific acute disorders, so malaria, by the action of its toxines, as well as by the debility it produces, may be responsible for an attack of insanity. In the febrile stage I have seen patients, who were at first in a condition of delirium, gradually pass into a condition of maniacal excitement with hallucinations which lasted from a few days to a week or more after all fever had passed off. The maniacal condition is certainly the most common, but I know of one or two cases where, after a chronic course of fever lasting off and on for some months, the patient has, apparently quite suddenly, passed into a semi-stuporose condition and wandered away from home and, when found about a month later, hundreds of miles perhaps away from his own village, has been in a state of bewilderment as regards his surroundings, and his mind a complete blank from the day of his leaving up to the time when he was found.

The maniacal condition is probably directly due to the action of malarial toxines and improves rapidly upon treatment with quinine, while the stuporose condition approximates more closely to an exhaustion psychosis and calls for rest, tonics and a full nourishing dietary. Saline purges are useful in either type of case, aiding the elimination of the toxines from the blood. A form of "exhaustion insanity" also occurs at times after malarial attacks and, owing to the delay in bringing such cases for treatment, the majority are practically received into the asylum in a demented condition.

As a rule the prognosis is good in the maniacal or stuporose cases, but in the cases approximating to an exhaustion psychosis it is by no means favourable as regards recovery of mentalisation.

III.—Sunstroke and Insanity.

Sunstroke is perhaps the commonest reason, given by relatives, for an attack of insanity, but in the vast majority of cases such a statement needs qualification. Sunstroke alone would hardly suffice to cause insanity, and in the greater number of such cases careful enquiry elicits a history of alcoholic abuse which is undoubtedly a potent factor in the production of insanity. Moreover it is people of these habits who are most liable to be exposed to heat as well as to suffer from its results.

The cases of insanity from sunstroke alone are practically confined to that type of "insolation" described by Sir Patrick Manson, in his work on Tropical Diseases, under the term of "Sun traumatism."

In such a condition the patient becomes ill while actually exposed to the sun's rays. A certain number of such cases may even die suddenly from cardiac syncope, but others are seized with high fever, vomiting, headache and delirium, with a full quick pulse and intolerance of light, sound and movement. A lengthy period of debility and ill-health may occur after such a seizure, and such cases are extremely liable to be affected with loss of memory, tremor, deafness, amblyopia, constant headaches, and occasionally epilepsy and insanity are said to occur.

In practically all such cases after recovery the least exposure to heat and sun is liable to bring on a recurrence, while if the smallest quantity of alcohol be imbibed a condition of acute drunkenness is aroused.

Three types of this mental affection are described by Major Ewens.

1. A form approximating closely to organic dementia, where after recovery the patient is left foolish, timid

and depressed, incapable of doing his former work, irritable and passionate, and peculiarly susceptible to the action of alcohol or to exposure to the sun. The symptoms vary from practically complete dementia up to little more than a change of temperament and a liability to intense fits of passion.

2. A form characterised by changes practically limited to one only of the mental functions, such as pronounced amnesia, or a social or a moral change. In all such cases sudden exacerbations of the mental symptoms are likely to occur and to be associated with loss of sight or hearing, severe headaches and paræsthesia along the distribution of nerves arising from certain parts of the spinal cord, this latter symptom being especially prominent when the back has been exposed to the sun, as occurs at times when, during a day's shooting, the man is crawling along, stalking his game.

3. A post-febrile psychosis occurring after the acute symptoms of "sun traumatism" have subsided. Such patients are, as a rule, excited and restless and are troubled with hallucinations and delusions of persecution. As a result of the delusions they are irritable and passionate, unruly and at times even homicidal. Such cases usually recover after some months, but never seem quite to regain their former mental equilibrium, being constantly moody and irritable.

IV.—Influenza and Insanity.

The toxines formed by the Influenza Bacillus seem especially prone to affect the nervous elements of the body, and very few people indeed pass through an attack without revealing some more or less marked mental or nervous symptoms. As a rule the condition is one of mild depression with irritability and loss of capacity for work. Headaches and neuralgias may be a constant source of worry to the patient, while insomnia may call for immediate treatment to avert a mental breakdown, and neurasthenia is at times seen as a sequel to an attack of influenza.

The severity of the mental symptoms is by no means in proportion to the severity of the attack of influenza, a very mild attack apparently often producing profound mental derangement, especially in persons with a tainted heredity.

Where the mental symptoms arise during the febrile stage of the disease, the condition generally is one of acute excitement and of a maniacal type; the most usual form, however, is where convalescence is apparently established, and after some weeks have elapsed since the abatement of the fever melancholic symptoms supervene.

Symptoms.—In the maniacal type the patient becomes noisy and restless and troubled by hallucinations both of sight and hearing. Occasionally the excitement may be so intense as to necessitate his removal to an asylum. As a rule such cases pass after a time into a depressed condition, during which refusal of food may call for tube feeding, and from this depressed condition the patient gradually returns to his normal mentalisation.

In the post-febrile type the onset is often most insidious, and insanity may have been developing for some time before the relatives begin to suspect the true state of affairs. A history of insomnia is very common in such cases and, combined with anorexia, undermines both the mental and physical health. Work becomes a labour, and indolence and lethargy become marked characteristics of the patient. At this stage the patient is constantly depressed in the morning and suicidal feelings gradually force themselves upon him. If the condition progresses still further the patient passes into a condition of marked melancholia with pronounced hallucinations and delusions, in some cases of a hypochondriacal type, in others those of suspicion and persecution.

Treatment.—This resolves itself into the treatment of the physical disease which is detailed in any text book on Medicine, and the treatment of the mental symptoms which have already been described under melancholia and mania.

Prognosis.—Such cases usually recover quickly if treatment is begun early in the course of insanity; persistent auditory hallucinations however are a bad prognostic sign and should invariably make us guarded in our prognosis.

V.—Rheumatic Fever and Insanity.

Rheumatic Fever seems capable, like many other acute diseases, of causing mental symptoms and affecting the nervous tissues in a similar way to that in which it affects the other tissues of the body. That this is so, is not a matter of much wonder when we consider the results of recent investigations both into rheumatic fever and into the causation of insanity. The probability is that the streptococcus described by Triboukt, Westphal, Wasserman, Poyntou, Paine and others and known as the "micrococcus rheumaticus" is capable of forming toxines which act on the nervous tissues, causing varied manifestations of insanity. Hence here again we are probably dealing with a bacterial toxæmia, and have yet another reminder of the importance of investigating closely the origin of our cases so that we may the better be enabled to treat them successfully. Moreover, apart from actual insanity, after an attack of rheumatic fever the patient may occasionally be found completely altered either mentally or morally, and Savage in writing on this very subject states: "We have met with several patients, mostly women, who have ceased to perform their domestic duties, and have caused family discord in consequence of their changed habits, the industrious mother becoming indolent and negligent of her duties. It is certain too that some persons, who before rheumatic fever were sober and truthful, after it become intemperate and untruthful."

The mental disorder varies both as to the time of its appearance and its manifestations. The fever may pass on to acute mania, or mental symptoms develope at a later stage of the disease. In these latter forms either melancholia or mania may be present, but mania is the more common. Where cardiac complications are present, however, the type of insanity is largely affected by them, mania being more common with aortic and melancholia with mitral disease.

Treatment.—This turns on general lines both as regards the physical and mental conditions, but the probability of cardiac disease should never be forgotten in these cases, and a careful search should always be made for valvular lesions.

Prognosis.—The prognosis, as regards the mental symptoms, is always hopeful in these cases as most cases make a good recovery ; a recurrence, however, is always to be feared when any subsequent attack of rheumatic fever occurs.

VI.—Heart Disease and Insanity.

Except for the changes caused in the blood supply to the brain little or no effect is produced by valvular lesions. Anxiety and restlessness are common concomitants of aortic insufficiency, and insomnia may lead to an attack of acute insanity in a person suffering from any form of valvular disease. As a rule cases of aortic insufficiency, with a low blood pressure, usually suffer from symptoms of mania or excited melancholia, while in cases of early mitral disease where the blood pressure is high the symptoms approximate more closely to those of acute melancholia, which is what one would expect from the state of blood pressure which is really the cause of the condition.

Prognosis.—The prognosis in such cases is far from hopeful.

VII.—Syphilis and Insanity.

The relationship of syphilis to insanity is at the present time a point of much discussion.

There is undoubtedly a great tendency among practitioners in India, whenever they meet with a mental disease whose origin is obscure, to put it down either to syphilis or drugs, especially one or other preparation of Cannabis Indica, and I would strongly protest against such action. Both these causes produce very distinctive features, if the mental condition be indeed due to them, and, unless these symptoms be present, I maintain that, even though a history of drug abuse or syphilitic infection be obtainable, it is wrong to enter either as an ætiological factor in the causation of the disease.

Cases of insanity, however, occur in which there can be no doubt as to the syphilitic origin of the disease. Thus a cachectic condition may be produced by the action of the poison on the blood forming tissues, arterio-sclerotic conditions may arise from its action on the blood vessels, or local or diffuse lesions of the brain and its membranes, such as gummata or sclerotic changes, may ensue.

Like many other diseases syphilis does not affect all its victims in a similar manner, thus in one case the viscera may be attacked, while in another the vascular or nervous elements may be affected. Strangely enough too persons with a neurotic heredity seem by no means prone to be affected mentally by the syphilitic poison, in fact the experience of well-known authorities seems to point in the opposite direction.

Savage has drawn up the following scheme of the relationship between syphilis and insanity :—

1. Insane dread of syphilis.
2. Insane dread of results of syphilis.
3. Syphilitic fever, delirium and mania.
4. Acute syphilis leading to mental decay.

5. Syphilitic cachexia, dyscrasia and mental disorder.
6. Syphilitic neuritis (optic), suspicion and mania.
7. Syphilitic ulceration, disfigurement and morbid self-consciousness.
8. Congenital syphilis, cranial, sensory and nerve tissue defects.
9. Congenital syphilis, epilepsy and idiocy.
10. Infantile syphilis acquired.
11. Constitutional syphilis, (1) vascular or fibrous; (2) Epilepsy; (3) hemiplegia; (4) local palsies; (5) general paralysis, spinal (spastic and tabetic), peripheral.
12. Locomotor ataxy (1) with insane crises; (2) with insane interpretation of ordinary symptoms.

The first class comprises those who have an insane dread of syphilis, and who may in fact never have had the disease in any form. It is in fact an obsessional insanity and has been termed "syphilophobia." The patient spends his days washing and scrubbing himself and his belongings, searching his body for symptoms of syphilis, and worrying himself into a depressed and delusional state in which suicide is common. This type is fairly common among Europeans and Eurasians, but I have never heard of a case in an Indian.

The second class of this affection is also to be seen in Europeans and Eurasians, and leads to very much the same sort of symptoms. Besides being suicidal, however, such cases are liable to commit homicide, a husband perhaps killing his wife and child in the belief that he has given them the disease also.

The third type is generally of short duration, lasting two or three months, and is practically an attack of acute mania. The action of the syphilitic toxines, combined perhaps with a careless administration of mercury, as is the common practice of so many hakims, leads in many cases to a cachectic condition with trophic changes in the brain and subsequent insanity. This may be either melancholia or mania at its onset, but, as a rule, such cases tend to rapid dementia.

In other cases where the syphilitic lesions attack the face, the patient may become hypersensitive, imagine people abuse and avoid him, and finally pass into a typical state of delusional insanity.

Congenital syphilis may lead to any of the conditions treated of under idiocy and imbecility, and to these (Chap. XVIII) I would refer my readers.

True cerebral syphilis as a rule developes within 10 years of the primary infection, and the greatest danger of its developing is during the first three or four years after infection, the risk decreasing with each additional year. The patient may at times simply show a gradual and progressive mental decay, passing finally into a condition of profound dementia, but, as a rule, maniacal symptoms are manifest, at first with probably delusions of grandeur or at times of persecution. Such patients are, as a rule, very irritable and liable to sudden and violent outbursts of passion. The majority of such cases sooner or later join the class of those suffering from organic dementia. G. P. I. and locomotor ataxy are entered here both because of being in Savage's Scheme, and also because, in spite of the work done by Ford Robertson and others, the generally accepted view among alienists nowadays is that these two conditions are the terminal results of syphilis, and may appear after all other symptoms, even reaction to Wasserman's test, have disappeared. The matter is, however, still under discussion.

Treatment.—This should invariably be begun early. Injections of Salvarsan should be tried in all cases where no sign of dementia has yet appeared. Where any sign of dementia is manifest, potassium iodide, combined at times with mercury, is the only practical method of treatment, and large doses should be given, 20—30 up to 40 or even 60 grains thrice daily if the patient can stand it. In some cases where the vascular system is specially affected iodide of sodium is a better preparation to exhibit as the potassium salt tends to increase arterial tension.

Mercury may be given, as the liq. hydr. perchlor., or in the form of an inunction, and where headache is severe shaving the scalp and then rubbing in mercurial ointment often produces wonderful results.

During treatment the general diet and health should, of course, be looked after and special care taken in the cleaning of the patient's mouth, which should be done after every meal and a gargle of chlorate of potash used at the same time.

The treatment should be continued for at least a year after the cessation of all symptoms, and the patient should be carefully informed as to the extreme necessity of his leading a regular temperate life in the future and going through a three months' course of treatment yearly for at least three years.

Prognosis.—In cases due to gummata and where treatment has been begun early the prognosis is decidedly hopeful, but in other cases, especially where there are marked depression and delusions, the prognosis is by no means good, only about 25 per cent. making any sort of recovery and most of them relapsing sooner or later.

VIII.—Chorea and Insanity.

There is no special type of insanity peculiarly characteristic of chorea or which can be properly called "choreic insanity," but chorea and insanity are really very closely allied. In nearly every case of chorea there are some symptoms of mental disturbance, in some cases mere apathy and listlessness with slight loss of memory, symptoms so mild indeed that they often escape unnoticed, all attention being directed to the severer physical manifestations. Sir William Gowers too has shown that chorea is much more prevalent among those with a neurotic heredity, and that insanity may either precede or follow after the physical symptoms.

Ætiology.—Mental symptoms are much more common in adults affected by chorea than in children suffering from the same complaint, and usually occur in persons with a tainted heredity. Women who develope chorea during pregnancy are especially liable to mental derangements. Chorea, however, rarely occurs primarily in an adult, most of such cases having already suffered from the disease in childhood, except in that type of the disease known as Huntington's chorea.

Symptoms.—Various types of insanity may be associated with chorea.

1. *Choreic mania.*—This as a rule occurs in the early stages of the physical disease, generally in the second or third week. The restless agitation of the chorea passes gradually into a condition of excitement, accompanied by loss of self-control and impulsiveness. Sleep is invariably markedly disturbed in such cases, and a condition of great confusion is present, while both auditory and visual hallucinations are common. At times such cases may be extremely affected mentally, with raised temperature, restless excitement, absolute insomnia and refusal of food, and such patients are very liable to die from exhaustion and syncope.

2. *Choreic stupor.*—This commonly occurs later in the course of the physical disease, the general lassitude and confusion common in choreic cases becoming gradually more profound until it merges into a condition of stupor.

3. *Choreic delusional insanity.*—In chronic cases of chorea a condition of mental derangement with delusions of persecution and suspicion at times arises.

4. *Huntington's chorea* (hereditary progressive chorea) was noted first by Huntington in 1872.

It is a hereditary condition tending to be transmitted through several generations, and usually affects people between 30 and 45, *i.e.*, it is a disease of middle life. It affects the sexes equally and may be transmitted either by father or mother. It is a progressive and incurable condition accompanied by increasing mental deterioration which finally ends in dementia. The muscles of the head and upper limbs are first affected, but gradually the whole of the voluntary muscles become implicated by the movements which, though at first fairly well under control, gradually become more extensive and less controllable. The early mental symptoms of general apathy and listlessness soon pass into a condition of profound depression, marked by occasional outbursts of irritability and anger, which sooner or later merges into a condition of complete dementia. Life is not shortened by this condition.

Treatment.—The treatment here should be on general principles. The diet should be liberal and nourishing, and meat should be avoided as much as possible. If food is refused forced feeding should be at once resorted to, and in severe cases stimulants should be given whenever the physical symptoms call for them. The bowels should be carefully looked to and kept rather on the loose side by means of salines or cascara. Sedatives are required for the insomnia and chloral hydrate is about the best in such cases where it can be safely used; failing chloral hydrate, paraldehyde or veronal are of great service.

Where the movements are violent and the patient restless or excited, care should be taken to prevent his being injured, and it is better to keep him on a mattress on the floor surrounded by other mattresses.

Prognosis.—Except for the acutely maniacal cases which often rapidly terminate fatally, the prognosis is as a rule good in the maniacal and melancholic forms of mental disorder, such cases recovering as a rule in a few weeks. In the stuporose form the prognosis should be more guarded as the duration is longer, and at times such cases pass into a condition of dementia.

Huntington's chorea is progressive and incurable. In cases where chorea supervenes on an attack of insanity, so far as I have seen the mental condition seems but little affected by the presence of the physical symptoms, but the choreic symptoms are as a rule chronic and incurable.

IX. Pregnancy and Insanity.

Insanity frequently occurs during the course of pregnancy, and generally partakes of a depressed delusional condition, though at times maniacal symptoms are met with.

The cases are divisible into two types, *viz.*—(*a*) Those occurring during the first four months of pregnancy; (*b*) those occurring during the later months.

In the former type of case recovery as a rule occurs before the time of parturition, and in the latter recovery ensues several months after parturition. In neither case is recovery accelerated by inducing premature labour, and therefore this should never be attempted for mental symptoms alone.

X. Menstruation and Insanity.

During menstruation women are much more liable to suffer from insanity and various neuroses. An enquiry among female criminals in Europe elicited the fact that in a very large percentage indeed the crime was committed during a menstrual period. Most cases too of kleptomania, and other impulsive insanities among women, occur during the process of menstruation. In asylums too in the female sections maniacs are always more maniacal, melancholiacs more depressed during a menstrual period.

This point is well worth remembering as it has important medico-legal bearings.

CHAPTER XX.

PHYSICAL CONDITIONS LIABLE TO COMPLICATE INSANITY.

The insane are as liable to physical disease as the saner portion of the community, and it is not proposed here to go into a disquisition on medicine and surgery, though as from 15-20 per cent. of an asylum population is constantly in hospital, ample scope might perhaps be found for it, but merely to bring to notice certain conditions which seem especially liable to affect the inhabitants of asylums and others who suffer from mental derangement.

I.—Hæmatoma Auris.

This condition, which is also known as Othæmatoma or the Insane Ear, has given rise to much discussion concerning its cause, and three distinct opinions are mooted on this point. Some say it is simply due to an effusion of blood between the cartilage of the ear and its perichondrium, such as at times occurs in those who play Rugby football, others affirm that it is primarily due to trophic changes in the cartilage which render hæmorrhage more likely on account of the weakening of the arterial and venous walls, while others say it is due to changes in the blood. Personally I strongly favour the second view in most cases, for I have seen this condition in cases where little or no injury could have been sustained, and its prevalence among the chronic insane and general paralytics, where trophic changes are so common and forced feeding seldom if ever required, strongly supports this theory. I have undoubtedly seen a few cases where the first theory is tenable, but, as a rule, the injury received is so slight that no result would have ensued had the ear been in a healthy condition, the injury perhaps consisting in the patient's rubbing the ear with his hands or even against the pillow. The third theory I think is ruled out of court by the fact that the condition is more commonly unilateral, whereas if due to blood changes the opposite would be the case.

Symptoms.—When first seen it appears as a smooth tense swelling limited to the cartilaginous parts of the ear and occupying the anterior or outer part of the auricle. It is acutely tender to the touch and causes much discomfort to the patient. If left untreated the hæmatoma may rupture or become slowly organised, but in either case much wrinkling and deformity of the ear ensues.

Treatment.—I have heard some teachers recommend cutting down and evacuating the contents of the cyst, but by far the greater number of authorities advocate the use of a blistering fluid and strongly deprecate the use of a knife. Certainly what I have seen of such cases has made me a strong adherent of this last method, for I have never seen a case where the knife has been used recover without marked deformity of the ear remaining, whereas if blistering fluid be applied early the swelling subsides, and in the large majority of cases very little puckering ensues.

II.—Lesions of the Osseous System.

Fractures are extremely liable to occur among the insane, not only from their being more liable to receive injuries, but also from injuries often producing fractures in the insane, which in the sane would merely cause a contusion or sprain.

Extreme excitement, restlessness, irritability and lack of cognition of place are the main reasons rendering the insane more liable to receive injuries, while a deficiency of reflex action, delayed reaction as it is sometimes termed, as well as nervous lesions and changes in the osseous system, render a slight injury much more likely to cause a fracture in an insane than a sane person. Insane people as a rule show a much larger percentage of cases of syphilis than does the normal population, and the presence of gummata in many of such cases has a distinct effect in rendering fractures more probable, especially when combined with the mental and nervous conditions already enumerated. In cases of chronic insanity there is a tendency to absorption of the internal parts of the bones, especially of the ribs, and in time not only may the inner parts be absorbed, but even the inner surface of the external parts of the bones may become affected and riddled with cavities, the bone absorbed being replaced with a fatty material. As can readily be imagined bones thus affected are brittle and easily fractured, and even attempts at artificial respiration may produce serious injury in such cases, no matter how carefully the manipulations are carried out. Chemical examination of such bones has shown a relative increase of organic matter to earthy constituents, and a decrease of the proportion of lime to phosphoric acid.

As a general rule, in spite of incessant restlessness and movement in many of the cases, fractures among the insane show just as good results as among the ordinary population, and there is no very marked increase in the number of ununited fractures in an asylum when compared with the statistics of other hospitals.

III.—Wounds, Ulcers, &c.

Owing to trophic changes, the habit so common among many of the insane of constantly picking at the skin or hair, and the disregard of cleanliness displayed by so many asylum patients, who plaster themselves with excreta, etc., etc., ulcers are common and any small wound or scratch is very liable to suppurate. It is practically impossible too to keep a surgical dressing applied for any length of time, for the patients promptly tear them off on every opportunity, and, scratching the wound, not only aggravate the condition but carry the sepsis to other parts of the body and in this way extensive glandular suppurations may result.

Cases of stupor or dementia require constant attention on this account, for such cases, as a rule, are indifferent to what settles on them, and any slight wound or abrasion is liable to become not only septic but swarming with maggots for this reason.

Curiously enough severe surgical cases among the insane generally run a more favourable course than minor ailments, probably owing to the greater pain and inconvenience compelling rest and attention, where a lesser hurt would be forgotten by the patient, or remembered only to be scratched.

I have got most excellent results of late in minor surgery among the insane by the use of iodine as a disinfectant. My habit is to use the Lin. Iodi on the unbroken skin around the wounds, while the wounds themselves are then washed either with boiled water or a weak boric lotion and then swabbed with Tr. Iodi, a simple asceptic gauze dressing being then applied. The dressing is performed twice daily, until convalescence is established when once a day suffices. In very severe cases it is carried out thrice a day. I have never seen a case of "iodism" arise from this method of treatment, and in all the results have been most satisfactory and to my mind better than would have been the case from ordinary dressings, and especially so in one or two cases of chronic tuberculosis.

A fact to be remembered is that an acute abscess, or carbuncle, or some similar condition may often seem the starting point of recovery in some of the acute insanities, probably owing to its effects on the leucocytic elements of the blood, and for this reason the subcutaneous injection of terebene is advocated by some authorities as a method of treatment in such cases.

IV.—MICRO-ORGANISMAL DISEASES.

Though much more immune to the results of changes of temperature than the sane community, the insane are, owing to weakened resistive powers, much more liable to suffer from micro-organismal diseases, and to these by far the larger number of deaths occurring annually in asylums is due.

Phthisis.—This disease seems gradually becoming less common in asylum practice owing to improved hygiene, etc. It is still, however, a source of much trouble at times, and its diagnosis in an insane patient, with little or no history, in the midst of the continual noise and clatter, as a rule present in most of the sections of an asylum, and perhaps with the patient himself constantly moving and chattering, is, as can be imagined, by no means an easy task.

"Why not examine his sputum?" I expect some of my readers will say, and that is undoubtedly done whenever possible, but to examine sputum you have to get it first, and in many cases this is by no means easy to accomplish. The microscopic examination of the sputum however is really our one means of diagnosis in many cases, and an invaluable aid too in all. The easy diagnosis of "Malaria" in any case of fever, especially with a young inexperienced Sub-Assistant Surgeon, is often a cause of many early cases of phthisis being overlooked, and this disease should always be kept in mind in such cases, or where there is progressive failure of health and nutrition, and a thorough examination made, not only of the patient but also of the sputum and the blood.

As a rule such cases run a rapid course and the prognosis is much less favourable than among the sane.

Pneumonia.—Is a fairly frequent condition and epidemics are very liable to occur in asylums, for the early diagnosis presents similar difficulties to those met with in tubercle, the patients expectorate on their blankets which get mixed by careless attendants, and some other patient, wrapping himself up, head and all, in the infected blanket, contracts the infection.

Many and varied are its modes of onset and symptoms. In some cases consolidation of the lung suddenly appears without any fever, cough or "rusty sputum," some cases remain undiscovered till thrombosis of the pulmonary artery carries them off, while others again have a typical acute attack, pass through the crisis, and apparently are convalescent with normal temperature, when suddenly death occurs apparently from collapse.

Extension to the pleura or pericardium has always to be looked for in these cases, as it is very liable to occur and equally liable to be missed owing to the difficulty of auscultating such cases.

The remarks anent the diagnosis of phthisis apply equally to these cases.

Dysentery and diarrhœa.—Except for malaria these are by far the most common type of micro-organismal infections in asylums as well as the most fatal. The dysentery, so far as my experience both at Home and in India goes, is mainly of the bacillary type, but it is always a critical condition to deal with and very often terminates fatally. The difficulty in treating such cases is enormous, as it is much more common among the more degraded patients who lie about naked, have no regard for cleanliness, but pass their motions anywhere and probably soil themselves and their food. Such patients too are frequently addicted to eating anything they can lay hands on, excreta, mud, sticks, leaves, pebbles are all one to them, and invariably find their way to their insatiable mouths unless a constant watch is kept over them. The difficulty therefore in treating such cases can be well imagined, but it can to a certain extent be overcome.

All such cases should be at once isolated and placed under the supervision of the very best attendants available, their excreta should be promptly cleared up and burnt by a sweeper especially detailed for the purpose, and the strictest supervision exercised over personal cleanliness and what the patients eat. It sounds simple but is really a most difficult task, though if it can be done the results of ordinary treatment are quite as satisfactory on the whole as among the rest of the population; such at least has been my experience during the last few months.

The number of cases of dysentery can be also enormously reduced if every latrine used by a dysenteric patient be burnt out with kerosine, and the barracks thoroughly disinfected with phenyle, while no one who has anything to do with such patients should have charge of anything connected with the feeding of the rest of the asylum.

Diarrhœa may be due to lack of proper secretion of the intestinal juices, causing an irritation of the intestinal tract by undigested food, or to irritation from some substance picked up and eaten during the day. Much the same remarks apply to it as to dysentery.

Malaria.—On the whole insane patients, in my little experience of them in India, are by no means more liable to be attacked by malaria than the rest of the community, in fact I should say they were rather less so, for in asylums due attention is paid to drainage, standing water is sprinkled with kerosine, and a weekly issue of quinine during the malarial season is the rule. The difficulty, however, is that notwithstanding all one's efforts a certain number of cases are bound to be overlooked at their commencement, and it is only when the patient is seriously affected and his constitution, at no time remarkably strong, beginning to be undermined, that the illness is discovered. Malaria too seems to take a firmer grip of the insane and to have a more weakening effect in such cases, with the result that though the percentage of deaths directly due to malaria may not be much larger than among the general population, yet indirectly it is the cause of a large number of deaths, patients, weakened by previous attacks of malaria, readily succumbing to other diseases such as pneumonia and dysentery.

Under the circumstances prophylaxis is our mainstay, and I would insist on the careful attention to efficient drainage, the application of kerosine oil to all stagnant pools around the house, and above all the prophylactic use of quinine in every case of insanity, whether a private patient or in an asylum, as the baneful influence of malaria on such cases is very great indeed.

V.—Menstrual Derangement.

One of the commonest physical derangements among insane women in Europe is some alteration in the menstrual function, amenorrhœa and dysmenorrhœa being very common in all types of insanity. In India, however, such derangement is by no means common, and it is worth while, I think, spending a little space in describing the reasons for it.

Let us consider first the menstruation prevailing among women resident in India. Dr. Chunni Lal, of the Agra Lunatic Asylum, tells me that menstruation varies among healthy Indian women according to their mode of living. The peasant or village girl menstruates first as a rule between 14 or 16 years of age, her periods correspond closely to a 4 weekly curve, and each period lasts about 4 days, rarely more; derangements of menstruation are rare in this class and generally tend towards suppression. In the city or town-bred female on the other hand, especially among the richer classes, the girls menstruate much earlier, generally well before 14 years of age, the periods are of longer duration (5-6 days) and are menorrhagic in their tendency. Menorrhagia is a common condition among this class of female, and is probably due to their environments and mode of living, their leading a life of luxurious ease in hot stuffy apartments, taking little if any exercise, eating plentifully of the richest of food and allowing their minds to run mainly on one subject—their duty to their husbands and the procreation of children.

Among Europeans and Eurasians in India the climate and the mode of living, etc., seems to have a similar effect on the womenfolk as is seen in the city or town-bred Indian women and menorrhagia is a common complaint, while amenorrhœa or dysmenorrhœa is comparatively rare, when we think of the frequency with which this latter condition prevails in England.

Having thus noted the conditions prevailing normally among women resident in India let us now glance at the condition of things existing at the present time in Agra Asylum.

Out of 58 native females under the age of forty, twelve suffer from disordered menstruation. Nine of these suffer from amenorrhœa, *viz.*, 6 cases of mania, 1 case of melancholia, 1 epileptic and 1 imbecile; of these nine, two cases are referrable to childbirth, *viz.*, 1 case of mania and 1 of epilepsy.

Three cases of menorrhagia are also present, *viz.*, 2 cases of excited melancholia and 1 of epilepsy.

Thus on the whole one cannot say there is much alteration from the normal, though perhaps the incidence of amenorrhœa is somewhat increased. This, however, may be explained by the very much larger percentage of lower class and peasant women in the asylum.

Out of 9 European and Eurasian women under forty, seven suffer from menorrhagia both as regards duration of flow and quantity of discharge, while two have normal menstruation—a result very different from our experience in English or Scotch asylums, but probably explicable by the very much larger percentage of chronic cases met with in Indian asylums.

If we may venture to generalise on such meagre figures, it would appear that menstruation in asylum cases in India, allowing for station of life and the results of climate, shows little, if any, departure from what might be expected among the sane population.

As a rule the appearance of a period tends to exaggerate the mental symptoms, and in cases of so-called "recurrent mania," menstruation seems at times to precipitate an attack, or if it occur during an exacerbation of the mental symptoms the flow is apt to be more profuse and of longer duration.

In one or two cases among native women I have elicted some history of deranged menstruation prior to the onset of the mental symptoms, but the reliability of such meagre information as one can gather on this point is always a matter for doubt.

CHAPTER XXI.

GENERAL TREATMENT.

THE ideal treatment of insanity really lies in the early recognition of the physical symptoms which precede the mental manifestations in so many cases. At the present time, however, our knowledge in this direction is so meagre that until definite mental symptoms arise the condition is, more often than not, allowed to pass unnoticed, either through the patients, being ignorant of their danger, not seeking medical advice till too late, or when they do consult a doctor giving him a misleading account of their symptoms, which, in the absence of friends to reveal changes in habits, temperament, etc., are quite liable to lead to a mistaken diagnosis.

Prophylaxis.—As a rule every case of incipient insanity presents signs of nutritional failure. The patient looks ill, his skin is dry and unhealthy in appearance, he is losing weight and troubled with dyspepsia, etc. Anæmia is usually present in such cases, and in certain of the toxic types it is highly probable that a hyperleucocytosis with an increase in the polymorphonuclear elements precedes the onset of mental symptoms. I can, however, find no literature on the point, and my own observations are too few to warrant a more definite statement.

When in addition to the above symptoms the patient is nervous and irritable, troubled with insomnia and has a high tension, rapid, irregular pulse, the possibility of an attack of insanity should always be kept in mind, especially where there is a neurotic taint in the family.

In such cases mental and physical rest are called for, and if the pulse be rapid and of high tension rest in bed is essential.

The diet should be liberal and nourishing, consisting mainly of milk and milk puddings. Tea, coffee, alcohol and butcher's meat should be strictly prohibited, while the patient should be encouraged to drink water freely between meals. Saline purges or enemata of normal saline solution should be regularly administered every third or fourth day. As a rule the symptoms subside rapidly under this treatment, but complete rest for at least two months should be insisted on.

Upbringing of children :—In children of a neurotic temperament much depends on the method of their upbringing. If such children are given a nourishing dietary, free from butcher's meat and tea and coffee, are encouraged to join in healthy outdoor exercise and their lives carefully regulated, the chances of their falling victims to an attack of insanity are greatly diminished.

General Treatment :—Where the mental disease is fully developed the treatment is purely and solely the treatment of the physical symptoms and those alone, for after all mental diseases are practically always an extension of physical disorders and are best dealt with on the lines of common sense and general medicine.

In early acute insanities the *condition of the alimentary tract* calls urgently for treatment. Carious teeth are invariably a source of chronic toxæmia and should be removed as soon as possible. Antiseptic gargles and mouthwashes, saline purges and the exhibition of salol are also called for in cases of bacterial infection to remove the cause of the toxæmia as far as possible. In most early cases of acute insanity anorexia is a marked symptom, and in such cases food should not be forced upon the patient, as there is generally a deficiency of the digestive secretions, and if 2 or 3 pints of milk be taken in the 24 hours one should rest content. When artificial feeding is necessary the food should always be digested beforehand, whether it be given by the œsophageal or the nasal tube.

Tube feeding :—(*a*) For the *feeding with the œsophageal tube* we require an œsophageal tube and funnel, which should have been previously thoroughly washed in warm water and then coiled up carefully in a large clean basin, a gag with its levers covered with India rubber or soft cloth is also necessary, a small jug of cold water, a jug containing the food readily digested, a small vessel of olive oil or glycerine, and a towel or waterproof sheet to prevent soiling the clothing. All these having been prepared the patient is placed in a semi-recumbent position and the sheet carefully wrapped round him; the operator then takes the gag, and, while an attendant steadies the head of the patient, gradually forces it between the teeth. Great care is needed during this part of the proceedings to keep the gag as nearly as possible at right angles to the plane of the teeth, for the least departure from this plane is apt to force a tooth out of the patient's jaw. The gag having been inserted, generally above the bicuspid teeth on either side, the attendant in charge of the head grasps the gag and is responsible for its being kept in position. The operator then, after lubricating the tube with oil or glycerine, passes it along the floor of the mouth and down the œsophagus for 17″ or 18″, when the escape of gas indicates the entry of the tube into the stomach. When this has occurred a small quantity of cold water is poured down to ascertain if the tube is clear, and thereafter the liquid food should be given as quickly as possible. The food should be carefully examined before administration and the operator must be certain that it is not too hot. After the food has been administered the tube should again be flushed with cold water and then rapidly and gently withdrawn, after which the patient should be placed in a recumbent position for about 15 minutes to avoid the occurrence of vomiting.

(*b*) When the *nasal tube* is resorted to practically the same appliances are required, except that a No. 12 or 13 nasal catheter with funnel is substituted for the œsophageal tube and no mouth gag is required. The patient should be in a sitting or semi-recumbent position, and his head steadied by an attendant. The nasal tube having been lubricated is then passed along the floor of one or other nostril, by no means always an easy matter, for a deflection of the nasal septum or an accumulation of dried mucus may completely obstruct the passage. During the passage of the tube the pharynx should be carefully watched for the reflex act of swallowing, when the tube can be passed into the œsophagus and thence into the stomach, otherwise the tube is liable to pass forward into the mouth or to curl up in the pharynx and cause choking. In the majority of cases choking occurs if the tube lodges in the pharynx, but in certain cases of stupor and G. P. I. the tube can even be passed into the trachea without causing any apparent inconvenience, and in such cases the only safeguard is to listen carefully to see that air does not pass through the tube during respiration. The rest of the operation is practically the same as with the œsophageal tube, except that during the act of withdrawal the tube must be firmly held between the finger and thumb of the right hand so that none of its contents can escape into the trachea.

Fever occurring in the insane is in India always a difficult question to deal with, the question of malaria being an ever-present one and having to be considered, as well as the question of the condition being purely a part of the insanity as we have seen often happens in many types of insanity. For this reason it is advisable, whenever possible, to make a blood examination in such cases, for though quinine is invaluable in its proper place, yet it is just as inadvisable to pile it unnecessarily into the insane as into the sane.

Hyperpyrexia as a purely mental manifestation rarely calls for treatment except in puerperal cases, and even there the condition is more probably due to physical than mental causes. When met with the ordinary treatment for such a condition, cold baths, sponging, etc., etc., is alone required.

Subnormal temperatures are liable to occur in stuporose and exhaustive conditions and require attention, calling for the application of hot bottles and extra blankets, and the administration of stimulants and hot milk, coffee, etc.

In acute toxic conditions, such as mania, acute melancholia and katatonia, any sudden drop in the temperature of the patient is always suggestive of the onset of typhoid symptoms and requires prompt attention, and the administration of stimulants, the rectal injection of warm normal saline solution and hot draughts of milk, etc.

Convalescence :—After the acute stage of any insanity is passed the patient should be encouraged to get outside, and endeavours made to stimulate his interest in his surroundings. Regular outdoor exercise should be arranged whenever possible, and regular work suited to his mental capacity should be provided as well as suitable amusements out of work hours. Walking exercise, tennis, football, hockey, cricket are all possible even in an asylum, for such patients are as a whole imitative, and if one or two can be got to make a beginning others in time join in, and the exercise, both mental and physical, does incalculable good if it be properly supervised and the patients are not allowed to become overfatigued. In epileptics especially regular exercise, and fairly heavy exercise too, is of the utmost benefit, as in this way energy is worked off in its proper channels and the fits are less liable to occur.

In restless violent cases we are often forced to adopt some one or other means of restraint. Various forms of appliances are in vogue, and each has some characteristic rendering it especially useful in a certain type of case.

The various forms most commonly in use are :—1. The padded room. 2. The sheet. 3. The strait-waistcoat. 4. The gloves or mittens. 5. Dr. Wolffe's "Protective Bed."

1. *The Padded Room.*—Although three or four of these are to be found in any asylum in Britain, I doubt if even one exists in India. Why this should be so was a constant puzzle to me on my first arriving in India, but I am bound to confess that I am now of opinion they can really be dispensed with out here. This sounds, perhaps, paradoxical after having stated that maniacal conditions are much more common in India than in Britain, but asylum conditions are totally different in the two countries. In an Indian Asylum if a patient shouts he is left alone, or at most a sedative is given if he requires it, and allowed to shout to his heart's content without the other patients being in any way affected. In Britain a similar patient seems to upset the whole place and has to be shut up in the padded room, where he can shout certainly, but no one hears the music but himself. The padded room is certainly useful in cases where patients go flinging themselves about, reckless of the wounds and bruises thus caused, and also in cases of severe epilepsy, but

I have found a thick layer of straw on the ground and a mattress on the top of that just as serviceable.

The chief objection to such an appliance out here is primarily perhaps the initial cost, but mainly the extreme rapidity with which the climate acts upon rubber, which would necessitate its being renewed at least every two years, if not oftener.

Such a room is essentially a small cell with floor, walls and door completely cushioned with thick rubber pads, and lighted by small "bull's eyes" high up and quite beyond the patient's reach. A small trapped pipe leads off from the centre of the floor to carry off urine, etc., when passed by the patient, and ventilation is usually arranged for either by Sherringham's valves or Tobyn's tubes. The door is a double one and the inner door is provided with a small flap shutter, fastening on the outside, for purposes of inspection.

2. *The Sheet.*—This appliance is rarely if ever used now. It consists essentially of a stout canvas sheet which is buckled to the bed, over the patient, and has, on its upper or outer surface, two arrangements like pockets into which the hands and arms of the patient are strapped. It is unnecessarily cumbersome and too forcible in its action, and has almost dropped out of use now on this account.

3. *The Straitwaistcoat.*—This is an excellent means of restraint especially in patients given to masturbation, to constantly picking at their hair or skin, or assaulting other patients. It has, however, to be used with caution as, though some cases seem never to mind it at all, others are liable to fret and worry

about it, and often half an hour in it reduces such patients to a condition of extreme exhaustion. Even in this latter class, however, its application is of great use, for the moral effect is marvellous, and gives one a means of stimulating their efforts at self-control. It must, however, be used with caution and only as a last resource when all efforts at persuasion have failed.

It consists of a canvas body fastening behind with three buckles, or else made in one piece like a jersey. From the body arms or sleeves come off which continue beyond the hands and terminate in blind extremities, their ends being sewn up. From the right sleeve a buckle and from the left a strap are led round the body and fastened behind the back, so that the arms are crossed on the chest. The special advantage of such an appliance is that the patient can get plenty of outdoor exercise even when under restraint.

4. *The Gloves or Mittens.*—These are invaluable in cases given to masturbation, or to picking or tearing their skin or hair. They consist of a pair of stout leather pockets placed over the closed hand of the patient and fastened round the wrist with a buckle. As the hand is closed nothing can be grasped, and so our object is, as a rule, achieved quite simply, and the patient's attention, being distracted by the condition of his hands, it is often quite possible to remove the gloves after a week or so without the patient returning to his former habits. A rough and ready imitation of these can be carried out with a couple of bandages or dusters arranged over the closed hand and tied round the wrist.

5. *Dr. Wolffe's "Protective Bed."*—This is a comparatively recent innovation, and has been much used in certain cases in the asylum at Basle. It is perhaps the best of all the methods at present in use, for instead of using forcible or mechanical restraints we are here employing what we may term "psychical restraint."

It consists essentially of an ordinary Lawson Tait Bedstead with the sides raised up twenty inches and the ends fifty inches, so that it somewhat resembles a gigantic child's crib. Inside these iron bars is attached wire netting and to the sides are hinged two frameworks of iron bars and netting which can be swung inwards and form a sloping roof over the patient. The lever mechanism controlling these flaps is of course outside the foot of the bed and inaccessible to the patient. The side flaps can be worked independently of each other and can be fixed in any position required. They can be turned right down outside the sides of the bed till they are in immediate contact with the legs of the bed, or raised till they meet and form an entire roof to the bed.

The bed, therefore, is intermediate between a padded room and a straitwaistcoat, and avoids most of the disadvantages of either. The patient remains in bed, in constant companionship and under constant supervision, and the disadvantages of the padded room are at once done away with. The patient enjoys the comparative use of all his limbs, can lie or sit at pleasure and move his hands and arms freely, and hence we have a great advantage over the straitwaistcoat. Of course a certain number of cases cannot be allowed even this small amount of freedom, but such cases are rare indeed in India, and such beds will, I hope, soon find their way into our asylums here.

The effect of these beds on patients in Basle Asylum is said to be extraordinary, not only on restless noisy cases, but in cases of delusional insanity and paranoia also, and in most, if not all, of the cases quoted the psychical effect was marked.

Before leaving the subject of restraint I would once more impress on my readers the necessity of avoiding it whenever possible. It should only be used as a last resource, and even then should never be applied as a punishment, but only with a view of preventing harm accruing to the patient and others. A little tact and patience go a long way in handling lunatics as in everything else, and where one man may be constantly resorting to some method of restraint, another man with a little tact and patience, a few chaffing remarks and kind interrogation or advice, may quiet some of the most turbulent patients and turn storm into calm, leaving the patient in entire possession of his liberty.

Hypnotism is, on the whole, best left alone in asylum practice and in our dealings with insane cases. It has been largely used on the continent in Europe, and occasionally good results have been obtained by it, but it tends to weaken volition and self-control still further, and I strongly warn the general practitioner against it, even though he may perhaps be an adept at it. In a certain few cases hypnotic suggestion may be at times employed with advantage, and I have occasionally employed it myself in one or two cases of delusional insanity with good results, but beyond this I have never gone for the reasons already given, and I strongly advise my readers to do the same. The difficulty of hypnotising a lunatic too is immense owing to the extreme difficulty there is in holding their attention, but it can be done if sufficient time and patience can be given to the task.

Serumtherapy.—Of late years the question of the bacteriological origin of many types of insanity has been a prominent one and many authorities have been investigating it with, on the whole, excellent results, and there can be no doubt that in the future serumtherapy will undoubtedly gain a wider scope in asylum practice.

As regards forms of insanity, such as mania and katatonia, in which at times a type of streptoccus has been found, polyvalent streptococcic vaccines have been used on one or two occasions with, it must be confessed, no very definite or marked results, but as the early administration of the sera or vaccines is half the battle in physical diseases, such as diphtheria, and the injections have in most cases been tried only on patients of some months' standing, such results are only to be expected, and judgment must be postponed till we hear the results of further investigation.

DRUG TREATMENT.

At present, therefore, our treatment is based mainly on common sense and general medical principles, but even here the knowledge of a bacterial toxæmia in many types of insanity is an excellent guide as to the lines on which our treatment is to be based, and in all such cases purgation and disinfection of the alimentary tract, the mouth, nose and nasopharynx are of great benefit. Calomel and saline purges are the best to use in such cases, and the occasional administration of large enemata is often of use in clearing the cæcum, especially if they are given through a long tube. Salol in 5 grain doses thrice daily is the best intestinal disinfectant available, but during its exhibition the urine must be carefully watched for signs of carboluria, and on its appearance the drug should be at once suspended; "medical izal" is another drug which may prove serviceable in such conditions.

For disinfection of the mouth and nasopharynx various gargles and nasal douches may be employed, but perhaps the best are dilutions of cyllin, boracic acid or potassium permanganate. The teeth should be carefully brushed after every meal, so as to keep the mouth as free from bacteria as possible.

Where the infection seems to come from the lungs but little can be done. Inhalations of eucalyptus, creosote, etc., probably never reach the site of infection, or if they do are so diluted that they have no effect, and the administration of creosote by the mouth is generally contraindicated by the presence of gastric derangement and the extreme probability of its causing nausea. Hence in these cases our attention must be mainly directed to building up the general health of the patient, strengthening his volition and self-control, and arousing an intelligent interest in his surroundings by means of suitable occupation and amusements. In puerperal conditions the uterus must be carefully examined and septic conditions treated.

Sedatives and Hypnotics.—Among a fair number of general practitioners and students I fear the idea largely prevails that in sedatives and hypnotics lies the main treatment for maniacal conditions and indeed for most forms of insanity, and nothing can be more erroneous, more harmful than such a belief, for though at times invaluable adjuvants in the treatment no patient can or should be treated with them alone.

Before giving such a drug various questions have to be decided. Is the drug likely to disorder other functions while mitigating insomnia and restlessness? Is the drug tending to restore the natural sleep habit or is it forming a bad brain habit that it will be difficult to overcome, *i.e.*, is it setting up a "drug habit"? How does the patient look and feel in the morning after the drug sleep, is he refreshed or otherwise?

It must also be remembered that what is pleasant for the patient is not necessarily good for him, and that in many cases to effect a cure we require especially to strengthen the volition, and we rather delay than hasten this object by the administration of hypnotics.

Another question has also to be settled and that is what type of drug is required, whether a pure hypnotic, a general sedative, a motor depressant or a combination of these. The reaction of patients to drugs varies widely, not only with the patient, but also at times in one and the same patient at different phases of his malady, and all this has to be carefully considered when we are going to order a sedative.

Roughly speaking these drugs may be divided into four classes according to their mode of action, (*a*) Pure hypnotics, such as paraldehyde and chloral; (*b*) Hypnotic sedatives, *e.g.*, sulphonal; (*c*) Sedatives both cerebral and spinal, such as the bromides and their combinations with hyoscyamus and cannabis indica; (*d*) Drugs which act by depressing the cortical motor centres, such as hyoscine. We must, therefore, also consider what class of drug is required before ordering blindly any sedative that comes into our mind, merely because we may have heard of its being useful in a case of insanity.

Opium and Chloral are drugs I have little liking for in mental cases. In cases of brain exhaustion small doses of opium and morphia are highly recommended by German and French authorities, and they undoubtedly have some good results to show. The risk of establishing a drug habit though is very great in such cases, and I would recommend every possible means being tried to induce natural sleep in such cases before a drug is resorted to, and even then opium or chloral would be the last I should have recourse to, paraldehyde being to my mind safer and better in every way. Opium, too, often seems to greatly increase the mental agitation of a patient, and this still further restricts its use. In fact I restrict its exhibition practically to cases of excited melancholia only, and in these I have often got wonderful results from a fairly small dose of some preparation of morphia.

Paraldehyde.—This is perhaps one of the most valuable and reliable hypnotics at the disposal of the alienist, and very rarely, indeed, is its administration followed by any discomfort, or even the feeling of heaviness so common after many other drugs of this sort. One great feature in its action is that the drug sleep gradually passes into natural sleep, and in many cases there is a distinct tendency to restore the "sleep habit."

Its use, however, has to be well considered as even it will not suit all cases and, as a rule, I make the pulse my guide under these circumstances. Thus in cases of insomnia with high arterial tension and rapid pulse rate, after all attempts at producing sleep by purgation, hot bottles, etc., have failed, paraldehyde in 2—3 drachm doses is by far the best drug we have. Where the arterial tension is low, however, such a dose would be worse than useless, tending rather to exaggerate the condition, and in such cases 10—15 minim doses of paraldehyde, or *sulphonal* grs. xx, or *trional* or *veronal* grs. x are rather indicated. In cases of extreme violence a cortical motor depressant is essential and here *hyoscine* is invaluable, $\frac{1}{200}$ — $\frac{1}{70}$ of a grain being injected subcutaneously. If, however, the violence be continuous then *sulphonal* or a combination of it with the bromides is indicated, being given frequently and in comparatively small doses.

Hyoscine and hyoscyamine must be given with care, and as a rule are best left alone, especially in acute cases, for there is always danger of their causing syncope. In such cases, too, especially in educated persons, I have seen vivid hallucinations of sight caused by these drugs. Consequently our administration of these preparations should be mainly restricted to cases of chronic insanity accompanied by extreme violence.

The bromides are often of great use, especially in those forms of insanity where there is marked depression and restlessness. In such cases the dose must be large (60 grains thrice daily as a rule), the patient practically being kept under the influence of the drug for some days and roused at periodic intervals to take food.

In epileptic cases, too, bromides are our chief resource, and by their constant exhibition we can generally greatly diminish both the number and severity of fits. Recently attempts have been made to increase the absorption of bromide by the tissues by means of reducing the chlorides present in food, etc. A special diet was drawn up whereby the chlorides naturally present were reduced to a minimum, and the results are said to have been very successful. I have tried substituting bromide for the sodium chloride usually added to the diet to see if any increased effect would be obtained, and as already stated (Chap. XVI) the results have been most satisfactory.

Sulphonal, Trional and Veronal are very similar drugs. Sulphonal is slow but cumulative in action and should be given at least five hours before its effects are desired, or else should be combined with some other drug such as potassium bromide. Owing to its cumulative action one dose often produces a good sleep on two consecutive nights. It is by no means a "safe" hypnotic, as so many of the laity fancy, for though some seem able to take it with impunity, others reveal a marked idiosyncrasy for it and symptoms of poisoning occur. Muscular weakness with inco-ordination of speech and action, vomiting and other gastric disturbances are common in such cases, and hæmatoporphyrinuria practically invariably occurs, which is a serious condition and death often follows in a few weeks. Sulphonal, therefore, must be administered with caution and never continuously, and such patients should be carefully watched and the bowels opened daily, by aperients if necessary.

Trional is more rapid in its action than sulphonal and acts best in aged patients. Its bad effects are similar to those of sulphonal but less common and milder as a rule.

Veronal is more uncertain but acts well and rapidly in some cases. It is useless in insomnia due to pain. Its exhibition too requires the greatest care and supervision to prevent poisoning.

Isopral has but recently been brought into use. It belongs to the chloral group and is a useful auxiliary to chloral. It is taken readily by patients and seems to produce a natural sleep without producing unpleasant symptoms. The dose is from 10—15 grains.

THYROID TREATMENT.

Thyroid treatment has of late come into prominence as a drug for insane patients of various types, and not only in cases where the condition is due to disease or derangements of the functions of the thyroid gland. It was first administered for the sake of the slight febrile attacks which result from its administration, for it was noticed that many insane patients began to improve mentally, and finally made good recoveries, after similar febrile attacks arising naturally. In such cases as a rule I confine the patient to bed and give 30 grs. of the extract daily for a week or ten days. After three or four days the patient's temperature becomes slightly febrile rising to 99°—100°F., and remaining so for nearly a week when it returns to normal and remains there even if the drug be continued. Marked gastric derangement is caused by the drug, and nausea and vomiting occur readily during its administration. The pulse becomes rapid and irregular, and the arterial tension falls markedly, while there is a progressive fall in the leucocytosis and the polymorphonuclear elements may fall below 40 per cent. Headaches, rheumatic pains, muscular tremors, profuse perspiration and rapid loss of weight often accompany its administration, but as a rule can be alleviated by a mild purgative. It must be remembered that the administration of this drug tends to aggravate phthisical disease and it is, therefore, contraindicated in such cases.

Mentally its effects vary greatly in different cases, some becoming depressed, others maniacal and others again emotional. Dr. Bruce explains this by the fact that a course of thyroid frequently reproduces for a short time the earlier acute symptoms of the mental disease from which the patient suffered. The question of thyroid extract being a direct cortical stimulant is still an open one. Undoubtedly in many cases of early secondary dementia, especially after acute mania, marked mental improvement has occurred during the administration of thyroid, but the condition is as a rule found on close examination to be more a state of subacute excitement, and though possibly due to direct cortical stimulation by the thyroid, it is just as likely that the diminished leucocytosis may allow the persistent toxæmia, common in post-maniacal states, to gain the upper hand for the time being, and that the apparent improvement is really only a mild recurrence of the primary mania.

Thyroid should never be administered in acute cases, but only when the acute symptoms have subsided and the case has become subacute, perhaps stuporose, as when a patient after an attack of acute mania passes into a confused, stuporose condition. In acute cases as I have already stated the drug exaggerates the condition, either by acting as a direct cortical stimulant or by allowing a greater degree of toxæmia from its effects on the leucocytosis.

When administered continuously, whether in large or small doses, much precaution is always necessary. Such patients should always be confined to bed, for the risk of heart-failure is great, and the diet must be carefully regulated and consist mainly of milk and farinaceous foods. Occasionally a toxic condition is noticed with a rapid thready pulse, dry harsh skin and subnormal temperature, but a hot drink and the application of hot bottles soon relieves this. In every case the lungs should be carefully examined before a course of the drug is commenced for phthisical disease is invariably aggravated by its exhibition.

APPENDIX I A.

SCHEDULE I, ACT IV OF 1912.

FORMS.

(*See section* 96).

FORM 1.

Application for Reception Order.

(*See sections* 5 *and* 6).

In the matter of A. B. (1), residing , by occupation , son of ; a person alleged to be a lunatic.

To Presidency Magistrate, for [*or* District Magistrate of , *or* Sub-divisional Magistrate of *or* Magistrate specially empowered under Act of 1912 for].

The petition of C. D. (1), residing at , by occupation , son of in the town of [*or* sub-division of in the district of].

1. I am (2) years of age.

---

(1) Full name, caste and titles.

(2) Enter the number of completed years. The petitioner must be at least eighteen or twenty-one whichever is the age of majority under the law to which the petitioner is subject.

2. I desire to obtain an order for the reception of A. B. as a lunatic in the asylum of situate at(1)

3. I last saw the said A. B. at on the (2) day of

4. I am the (3) of the said A. B. [*or if the petitioner is not a relative of the patient, state as follows.*]

I am not a relative of the said A. B. The reasons why this petition is not presented by a relative are as follows : [*State them.*]

The circumstances under which this petition is presented by me are as follows : [*State them.*]

5. The persons signing the medical certificates which accompany the petition are(4).

6. A statement of particulars relating to the said A. B. accompanies this petition.

7. [*If that is the fact.*] An application for an inquiry into the mental capacity of the said A. B. was made to the on the and a certified copy of the order made on the said petition is annexed hereto.

---

(1) Insert full description of the name and locality of the asylum of the name, address and description of the person in charge of the asylum.

(2) A day within 14 days before the date of the presentation of the petition is requisite.

(3) Here state the relationship with the patient.

(4) Here state whether either of the persons signing the medical certificates is a relative, partner or assistant of the lunatic or of the petitioner and, if a relative of either, the exact relationship.

[*Or if that is the fact.*] No application for an inquiry into the mental capacity of the said A. B. has been made previous to this application.

The petitioner therefore prays that a reception order may be made in accordance with the foregoing statement.

(Sd.) C. D.

The statements contained or referred to in paragraphs are true to my knowledge; the other statements are true to my information and belief.

(Sd.) C. D.

Dated

APPENDIX I B.

Statement of particulars.

[*If any of the particulars in this statement is not known, the fact to be so stated.*]

The following is a statement of particulars relating to the said A. B.

Name of patient at length.

Sex and age.

Married, single or widowed.

Previous occupation.

Caste and religious belief, as far as known.

Residence at or immediately previous to the date hereof.

Names of any near relatives to the patient who are alive.

Whether this is first attack of lunacy.

Age (if known) on first attack..

When and where previously under care and treatment as a lunatic.

Duration of existing attack.

Supposed cause.

Whether the patient is subject to epilepsy.

Whether suicidal.

Whether the patient is known to be suffering from phthisis or any form of tubercular disease.

Whether dangerous to others and in what way.

Whether any near relative (stating the relationship) has been afflicted with insanity.

Whether the patient is addicted to alcohol, or the use of opium, ganja, charas, bhang, cocaine or other intoxicant.

[The statements contained or referred to in paras. are true to my knowledge. The other statements are true to my information and belief.]

[*Signature by person making the statement.*]

APPENDIX II.

FORM 3.

Medical Certificate.

(*See sections* 18, 19).

In the matter of A. B. of (1) in the town of [*or* the sub-division of in the district of] an alleged lunatic.

---

(1) Insert residence of patient.

I, the undersigned C. D., do hereby certify as follows :

1. I am a gazatted medical officer [*or* a medical practitioner] a holder of (1) [*or* declared by Local Government to be a medical officer under Act of 1912]

and I am in the actual practice of the medical profession.

2. On the day of 19 at (2) in the of [*or* the sub-division of in the district of [separately from any other practitioner] (3), I personally examined the said A. B. and came to the conclusion that the said A. B. is a lunatic and a proper person to be taken charge of and detained under care and treatment.

3. I formed this conclusion on the following grounds, *viz.* :—

(*a*) Facts indicating insanity observed by myself, *viz.*:—

(*b*) Other facts (if any) indicating insanity communicated to me by others, *viz.* :—*Here state the information and from whom.*

(Sd.) C. D.

(*Designation as above.*)

---

(1) Insert qualification to practice medicine and surgery registrable in the United Kingdom.

(2) Insert place of examination.

(3) Omit this where only one certificate is required.

APPENDIX III.

FORM 2.

Reception order on petition.

(*See sections* 7, 10).

I, the undersigned E. F., being a Presidency Magistrate of [*or* the District Magistrate of *or* the Sub-divisional Magistrate of—*or* a Magistrate of the first class specially empowered by Government to perform the functions of a Magistrate under Act of 1912] upon the petition of C. D. of [1] in the matter of A. B., [1] a lunatic, accompanied by the medical certificates of G. H., a medical officer, and of J. K., a medical practitioner [*or* medical officer], under the said Act, hereto annexed, hereby authorise you to receive the said A. B. into your asylum. And I declare that I have [*or* have not] personally seen the said A. B. before making this order.

(Sd.) E. F.

(*Designation as above.*)

To[2]

---

(1) Address and description.

(2) To be addressed to the officer or person in charge of the asylum.

APPENDIX IV.

FORM 4.

Reception Order in case of Lunatic Soldier.

(*See section* 12).

Whereas it appears to me that A. B., a European, subject to the Army Act, who has been declared a lunatic in accordance with the provisions of the military regulations, should be removed to an asylum, I do hereby authorise you to receive the said A. B. into your asylum.

(Sd.) E. F.

(*Administrative Medical Officer.*)

To [1]

APPENDIX V.

FORM 5.

Reception Order in case of wandering or dangerous lunatics or lunatics not under proper control or cruelly treated (sent to an asylum established by Government).

(*See sections* 14, 15, 17).

I, C. D., Presidency Magistrate of [*or* Commissioner of Police for] [*or* the District

---

(1) To be addressed to the person in charge of an asylum duly authorised by Government to receive lunatic Europeans subject to the Army Act.

Magistrate of *or* the Sub-divisional Magistrate of *or* a Magistrate specially empowered by Government under Act of 1912] having caused A. B. to be examined by E. F., a Medical Officer under the Indian Lunacy Act, 1912, and being satisfied that A. B. [*describing him*] is a lunatic who was wandering at large [*or* is a person dangerous by reason of lunacy] [*or* is a lunatic not under proper care and control *or* is cruelly treated or neglected by the person having the care or charge of him] and a proper person to be taken charge of and detained under care and treatment, hereby direct you to receive the said A. B. into your asylum.

(Sd.) C. D.

(*Designation as above.*)

Dated the

To the officer in charge of the asylum at

APPENDIX VI.

FORM 6.

Same when sent to a licensed asylum.

I, C. D., [*as above down to* "care and treatment"] and being satisfied with the engagement entered into in writing by G. H. of [*here insert address and description*] who has desired that the said A. B. may be sent to the asylum at [*here insert description of asylum and name of the person in charge*] to pay the cost of maintenance of the said A. B., in the said asylum, hereby authorize you to receive the said A. B. into your asylum.

(Sd.) C. D.

(*Designation as above.*)

Dated the

To the person in charge of the asylum at

APPENDIX VII.

FORM 7.

Bond on the making over of a lunatic to the care of relative or friend.

(*See sections* 14, 15, 17).

Whereas A. B., son of , inhabitant of , has been brought up before C. D., a Presidency Magistrate for the town of [*or* Commissioner of Police for] [*or* the Magistrate of , *or* a Magistrate of the first class specially empowered under Act of 1912] and is a lunatic who is believed to be dangerous [*or* deemed to be a lunatic who is not under proper care and control or is cruelly treated or neglected by the person having the charge of him] and whereas I, E. F., son of inhabitant of , have applied to the Magistrate [*or* Commissioner of Police] that the said A. B. may be delivered to my care :

I, E. F., abovenamed hereby bind myself that on the said A. B. being made over to my care, I will have the said A. B. properly taken care of and prevented from doing injury to himself or to others: and in case of my making default therein, I hereby bind myself to forfeit to His Majesty the King-Emperor of India, the sum of rupees

Dated this day of 19

(Sd.) E. F.

(*Where a bond with sureties is to be executed add*)—We do hereby declare ourselves sureties for the abovenamed E. F. that he will, on the aforesaid A. B. being made over to his care have the said A. B. properly taken care of and prevented from doing injury to himself or to others; and in case of the said E. F. making default therein, we bind ourselves, jointly and severally to forfeit to His Majesty the King-Emperor of India, the sum of rupees

Dated this day of 19

(*Signature.*)

APPENDIX VIII.

FORM 8.

Bond on the discharge of a lunatic from an asylum on the undertaking of relative or friend to take due care.

(*See section* 33).

Whereas A. B., son of , inhabitant of , is a lunatic who is now detained in the asylum at under an order made by C. D., a Presidency Magistrate for the town of [*or* Commissioner of Police for] [*or* the Magistrate of , *or* a Magistrate of the first class specially empowered under Act of 1912] under section 14 [*or* section 15] of Act of 1912 and whereas I, E. F., son of , inhabitant of , have applied to the said Magistrate [*or* Commissioner of Police] that the said A. B. may be delivered to my care and custody :

I hereby bind myself that on the said A. B. being made over to my care and custody, I will have him properly taken care of and prevented from doing injury to himself or to others ; and in case of my making default therein, I hereby bind myself to forfeit to His Majesty the King-Emperor of India, the sum of rupees

Dated this day of 19

(Sd.) E. F.

(*Where a bond with sureties is to be executed add*)—We do hereby declare ourselves sureties for the abovenamed E. F. that he will, on the aforesaid A. B. being delivered to his care and custody, have the said A. B. properly taken care of and prevented from doing injury to himself or to others ; and in case of the said E. F. making default therein, we bind ourselves, jointly and severally, to forfeit to His Majesty the King-Emperor of India, the sum of rupees

Dated this day of 19

(*Signature.*)

INDEX.

A

Pages.

Abuse of drugs as a cause of insanity 34

Admission into Asylums, necessary procedures :—
- on petition of patient himself 3
- on petition of relatives 3
- of persons under Army Act 5
- of wandering or dangerous lunatics .. 5
- of lunatics ill-treated or not properly cared for 6
- after an inquisition under Chap. IV or V of Act IV, 1912.. 7

Æstheticism 52

Agglutinines 31, 35, 41, 62, 63, 92

Albuminuria (*see* Urine,) excretion of, in insanity).

Alcohol, insanities due to 43, 204
- varying effects of .. 205
- Craig on alcoholism .. 206
- ætiology 206
- (*a*) Acute intoxication .. 207
  - symptoms, physical 207
  - mental 207
  - treatment 207
- (*b*) Delirium tremens 43, 208
  - symptoms, physical 208
  - mental .. 208
  - diagnosis 209
  - treatment 209
  - prognosis 210
- (*c*) Mania à potu .. 210
  - ætiology 210
  - symptoms, physical 210
  - mental .. 211
  - diagnosis 211
  - treatment 211
  - prognosis 212
- (*d*) Chronic alcoholic insanity 43, 212
  - ætiology 212
  - symptoms, physical 212
  - mental 214
  - diagnosis 215
  - treatment 216
- (*e*) Dipsomania .. 44, 217

Alcoholism, a symptom of insanity .. 159, 206

Alexines 62

Alimentary tract, disorders of 60, 322
- treatment of .. 322

Pages.

Alternating insanity (*see* Folie Circulaire).
Amentia (*see* idiocy).
Anæmia and insanity,—
in exhaustion insanity 129
in acute melancholia 144
in chronic metabolic toxæmia 159
in excited melancholia 163
Antitoxic sera in G. P. I. 254
Appetite in acute insanity 61
Arterial tension (*see* Blood Pressure).
Atrophy of hemispheres 78
Attendants, servants of p.'s relatives 2
Attention 51, 72, 160
Aura in epilepsy .. 233
Autointoxications causing insanity, Macpherson's classification of .. 30

B

Bacteria in the blood 31, 63, 92
Bacteria in the mouth and nasopharynx 84
in the alimentary canal 31, 84
Bacterial examination of blood 31
of gastric contents .. 84
Bacterial toxæmias, insanities due to 41
Baths, hot 57
Bhang (*see* Indian Hemp).
Blood, coagulation of .. 84
hæmolysis 84
leucocytoses (*see* Leucocytosis).

Pages.

micro-organisms in 31, 63
agglutinines in 31, 35, 41, 62, 63, 92
alexines in 62
Blood pressure, as a cause of insanity 35
its relation to sleep .. 57
in nervous derangements .. 58, 64
in insanity due to brain anæmia 138
in acute melancholia 41, 143
in delusional insanity 154, 155
in chronic metabolic toxæmia .. 159
in excited melancholia 163
in folie circulaire 178-182
in katatonia 185-187
in chronic alcoholism 213
in G. P. I. 248, 250, 251
Boils and acute insanity 66
Bone-marrow, red, — in states of hyperleucocytosis .. 64
Brain anæmia, insanity due to 40-138
ætiology 138
symptoms, physical 138
mental 139
treatment 140
Brain substance, gross lesions of 77
Brain lesions, insanity due to gross .. 40, 131
Brain habits 57
Bromides, in katatonia .. 187
in alcoholism .. 209

Pages.
in epilepsy 241
in G. P. I. 255
as general sedatives .. 336
Bromism 241
Bruce's classification of insanity 39

C

Cannabis Indica (*see* Indian Hemp).
Carbon bi-sulphide poisoning, insanity due to 44, 226
Carious teeth and insanity 60
Causation of insanity .. 29
common ideas on .. 29
toxic theory of .. 29
Macpherson's classification of toxæmias .. 30
hereditary predisposition 32
non-toxic causes .. 36
toxic causes 37
Certification of patient .. 11
grounds for 11
procedure in .. 12
Certificates of sanity .. 14
Charas (*see* Indian Hemp).
Child-marriages, a cause of insanity 33
Chloral as an hypnotic .. 334
in alcoholism .. 209
in epilepsy 242
Chlorides, in Urine (*see* Urine, excretion of).
Chloroform, psychoses due to 44, 225
Chorea, insanity due to .. 303
ætiology 303

Pages.
symptoms 303
1. Choreic mania 304
2. Choreic stupor 304
3. Choreic delusional insanity 304
4. Huntington's chorea .. 304
treatment 305
prognosis 305
Chronic metabolic toxæmia 41, 158
ætiology 159
symptoms, physical 159
mental 159
diagnosis 160
treatment 160
prognosis 160
Circular Insanity (*see* Folie Circulaire).
Circulatory system in insanity 64
Classification of insanity, Bruce's 39
Clinical examination of patient 93
Clinical Pathology :—
agglutinines .. 92
bacteria of mouth and stomach 84
coagulation of blood 84
hæmolysis 84
leucocytosis 85
temperature .. 83
Cocainism .. 44, 224
symptoms, physical 224
mental .. 224
diagnosis 225
treatment 225

Pages.

prognosis 225
Committee of persons .. 17
Committee of estate .. 17
Confusion, mental .. 45
Congestive seizures in G. P. I. .. 245, 251, 252
Consanguineous marriages, a cause of insanity .. 33
Convalescence after insanity 325
Cortex, pathological changes in cerebral 78
Cranial bones, pathological changes in 75
Cretinism 273
Criminal lunatics .. 22
Criminal responsibility .. 19
Curator Bonis (*see* Committee of Estate).

D

Defæcation, affected in insanity 70
Degenerations of nerve-cells 79-81
staining methods .. 79
fatty degeneration .. 79
simple atrophy .. 80
coarse granular degeneration 80
vacuolation of protoplasm 80
colloid degeneration 81
depigmentation and hyaline degeneration 81
finely granular degeneration 81
calcareous degeneration 81

Pages.

Degenerations of nerve-fibres 81
Degenerations of neuralgia 82
Degenerations of blood-vessels 82
Deglutition, impairment of 71
Délire de toucher et de doute 114
Delirium Tremens (*see* Alcohol, Insanity due to).
Delusions 48, 70, 153, 160, 164, 167, 169, 173, 185, 188, 190, 195, 201, 209, 214
Delusions and criminal responsibility .. 21
Delusional insanity 19, 21, 40, 55, 152
definition 153
ætiology 154
symptoms 154
physical 154
mental 155
diagnosis 158
treatment 158
prognosis 158
Dementia 279
(*a*) Secondary dementia 44, 280
ætiology .. 280
symptoms, physical 281
mental 282
treatment .. 285
(*b*) Organic Dementia 44, 285
ætiology 285
symptoms, physical 287
mental 287
diagnosis 287
treatment .. 287
prognosis .. 288

Pages.

Dementia præcox .. 152
Depression (*see* Melancholia).
Deprivation of special senses,
idiocy from .. 267, 274
insanity from 40, 139
treatment .. 140
prognosis 141
and criminal lunatics 22
Derangements of mentalisation 45
Detention under observation 6
Detention pending removal to an asylum 7
Diarrhœa in the insane .. 314
Difference in incidence and manifestations of insanities common to Europe and India 101
Digestive juices, failure of, in acute insanity .. 61
Diphtheroid bacillus, Ford Robertson's 65
Dipsomania (*see* Alcohol, Insanities due to).
Discharge from asylums :—
of boarders 8
of non-criminal lunatics by committee .. 9
of lunatics admitted on petition of relatives 9
of persons under the Army Act .. 9
on undertaking of a relative 9
after an inquisition under Chap. IV or V, Act IV, 1912 .. 10

Pages.

Drink and criminal responsibility 21
Drugs and insanity .. 43
Drugs in general treatment 331
Dura Mater, pathological changes in .. 75
Dysentery and the insane 314

E

Elevation 45
Emotions, disturbances of 54
Epilepsy 44, 228
ætiology 232
Bevan Lewis on .. 229
toxic origin of .. 230
heredity in 232
exciting causes .. 232
symptoms, physical 232
1. Grand mal .. 233
2. Petit mal .. 234
3. Jacksonian epilepsy .. 234
4. Status epilepticus .. 234
mental 234
Insanity associated with epilepsy .. 236
1. Epileptic idiocy 236, 237
2. Pre-epileptic insanity .. 236, 237
3. Epilepsie larvée 21, 236, 237
4. Post-epileptic insanity 236, 238
5. Chronic epileptic insanity 236, 239

Pages.

diagnoris .. 239
treatment .. 240
prognosis .. 242
Eroticism 52
Escape and recapture .. 10
Ether, insanity due to 44, 225
Evidence, expert .. 21
Excited Melancholia (*see* Melancholia).
Excitement 45
Excitement with confusion (*see* Mania).
Excitement, without confusion (*see* Folie Circulaire).
Exciting causes of insanity 34
Exhaustion, insanity due to 39-128
ætiology 128
symptoms, prodromal 128
physical .. 128
mental 129
treatment 130
prognosis 131
diagnosis 131

F

Family advice 27
marriage 27
mental and moral changes 27
upbringing of neurotic children 28
Feeding by tube, nasal .. 323
œsophageal .. 323
Fever and insanity .. 324
Feigned insanity .. 23
Folie circulaire .. 42, 177
ætiology 177

Pages.

(*a*) Stage of elevation :—
symptoms, prodromal 178
physical 178
mental 179
diagnosis .. 180
treatment .. 181
prognosis .. 182
(*b*) Stage of depression :—
symptoms, physical 182
mental 182
diagnosis .. 183
treatment .. 183
prognosis .. 183
Folie de doute 115
Fractures of bones in the insane 310

G

Ganjah (*see* Indian Hemp).
General paralysis of the insane (G. P. I.) 44, 244
incidence in India .. 244
definition 245
ætiology 246
Ford Robertson's bacillus .. 65-246
Symptoms 247
(*a*) Prodromal, physical 247
mental .. 247
(*b*) 1st Stage, physical 248
mental .. 252
(*c*) 2nd Stage, physical 250
mental .. 253

Pages.

(d) 3rd Stage, physical 251
mental .. 254
diagnosis 254
treatment 254
prognosis 256
General treatment of insanity 320
Glycosuria in insanity (see Urine, excretion of).
Grand mal 233
Gross brain lesion, insanity due to 40

H

Hæmatoma auris .. 308
ætiology 308
symptoms 309
treatment 309
Hæmopoietic system in insanity 61
Handwriting in insanity 54
Hallucinations 46, 70
aural 47
visual 47
auditory 47
olfactory 47
of sensation .. 48
in acute melancholia 145
in delusional insanity 156
in chronic metabolic toxæmia .. 160
in excited melancholia 164
in acute mania 167, 173
in katatonia 184, 188, 190
in hebephrenia .. 195
in insanity due to Indian hemp 201, 203

Pages.

in chronic alcoholism 214
in delirium tremens 208
in morphinism .. 222
in cocainism .. 224
Haschisch (see Indian Hemp).
Heart lesions, insanity due to 298
Heart lesions, valvular, in insanity 64
Hebephrenia .. 43, 191
definition 192
ætiology 192
symptoms, prodromal 193
physical 193
mental 194
diagnosis 195
treatment 196
prognosis 196
Hereditary predisposition to mental disease .. 31
its significance .. 32
its effect 32
its manifestations .. 32
Hyoscine and hyoscyamine as sedatives 335
Hyoscyamus in katatonia 191
Hyperpyrexia in insanity 324
Hypnotics in insanity .. 333
Hypnotism 330
Hysteria, ætiology .. 123
deviations from normal mentalisation .. 124
interparoxysmal psychoses .. 124
mental hysteria .. 125
postparoxysmal psychoser .. 125

Pages.

hysteroepilepsy 126
lethargy 126
suicide in 127
treatment 127
Hysterical psychoses .. 122

I

Idiocy and imbecility 44, 257
Ireland's definition .. 257
ætiology 257
symptoms, general .. 260
physical 261
mental 264
Types of idiocy:—
1. Genetous 267, 268
2. Mongolian 267, 268
3. Micro-cephalic 267, 269
4. Hydro-cephalic 267, 269
5. Hypertrophic 267, 270
6. Eclampsic 267, 270
7. Epileptic 267, 271
8. Paralytic 267, 272
9. Traumatic 267, 272
10. Inflammatory 267, 272
11. Syphilitic 267, 273
12. Cretinoid 267, 273
13. From deprivation of the special senses .. 267, 274
14. Shah Daula's mice 99, 268, 274
treatment 274
Illegal detention 10
Illusions .. 48, 167
Imbecility (*see* Idiocy).

Pages.

Impulsiveness 51
Impulsive insanities 20, 218
Incoherence 54
Inco-ordination 71
Indian hemp as a sedative in katatonia 191
as a cause of insanity 34
insanity due to 44, 197
ætiology 198
Symptoms:
(*a*) Acute cases:—
1. Acute intoxication 201
symptoms, physical 201
mental 201
treatment .. 202
2. Transitory excitement .. 202
symptoms, physical 202
mental 203
diagnosis .. 203
treatment .. 203
prognosis .. 203
(*b*) Chronic cases:—
symptoms .. 204
prognosis .. 204
Influence of a tropical climate upon Europeans 97
Influenza, mental derangements due to 294
symptoms .. 295
treatment .. 296
prognosis .. 296
Integumentary system in insanity .. 65, 129

Pages.

Intracranial tumours, insanity due to 286
Iodoform poisoning, insanity due to .. 44, 225
Isopral as an hypnotic .. 337

J

Jacksonian epilepsy .. 234
Jealousy 53

K

Katatonia .. 42, 183
    definition 184
    ætiology 184
    Symptoms: (*a*) Prodromal 184
      (*b*) Acute onset:—
        symptoms, physical 185
          mental .. 186
        diagnosis .. 186
        treatment .. 186
        prognosis .. 187
      (*c*) Stage of stupor:—
        symptoms, physical 187
          mental .. 188
        diagnosis .. 189
        treatment .. 189
        prognosis .. 189
      (*d*) Stage of excitement:—
        symptoms, physical 190
          mental .. 190
        diagnosis .. 190
        treatment .. 191
        prognosis .. 191
Kleptomania 20

Pages.

L

Lachrymal secretion in insanity 69
Lactation, a cause of insanity 34
Larvated epilepsy (*see* Epilepsie Larvée).
Lead poisoning, insanity due to 44-226
Leucocytes (*see* Leucocytosis).
Leucocytosis, an aid in detecting malingerers .. 23
Leucocytosis, general remarks on .. 35, 62, 85
    in non-toxic insanities 86, 129, 139
    in metabolic toxæmias 86
    in acute melancholia 40, 143
    in bacterial toxæmias 41, 87, 91, 161
    in acute mania 41, 87, 171
    in excited melancholia, 41, 87, 163
    in folie circulaire .. 42, 88, 178, 182
    in katatonia 42, 43, 88, 185, 187
    in hebephrenia 43, 90, 194
    in G. P. I. 90, 248, 250, 251
    in epileptics .. 91, 230
    in idiots and imbeciles 91
    in secondary dementia 91
    in delirium tremens 208

M

Malaria, insanity due to .. 191
Malaria in the insane 29, 315

Pages.

Management of property 16
Mania 41, 166, 168
 ætiology 168
 symptoms, prodromal 168
  physical 169
  mental 172
 diagnosis 174
 treatment 174
 prognosis 175
Mania à Potu (*see* Alcohol, Insanities due to).
Manio-depressive insanity (*see* Folie Circulaire).
Marriage and insanity .. 27
Masturbation 67
Medico-legal duties .. 1
Medico-legal References :—
 Act IV, Lunacy Act, of 1912 :—
 Admission into asylums 3—7
  on petition of p. himself 3
  on petition of relatives 3
  of persons under the Army Act .. 5
  of wandering or dangerous lunatics .. 5
  of lunatics ill-treated or uncared for .. 6
  detention under observation 6
  detention pending removal to an asylum 7
  admission after an inquisition under Chap. IV or V of Act .. 7
  discharge of lunatics 8—10
  n petition of p. himself 8

Pages.

 by the asylum committee 9
 of lunatics detained under petition of relatives 9
 of persons under the Army Act .. 9
 on undertaking of a relative 9
 of persons pronounced sane by an inquisition 10
 transfers from one asylum to another 10
 escape and recapture 10
 illegal detention .. 10
 management of property 16
 certification of patient 11
 grounds for 11
 modus operandi .. 12
 certificates of sanity .. 14
 criminal lunatics .. 22
 criminal responsibility 9—21
 insanities mainly involved in crime 19—21
 mania 19, 166, 173
 epileptic insanity 19, 21, 154, 228, 235, 237, 239
 delusional insanity 19, 21, 157
 alcoholic insanities 19, 205, 209, 210, 214
 puerperal insanity 19, 176
 acute melancholia 19, 146, 147
 amentia 19, 262, 266, 269, 271, 279

Pages.

dementia 20, 284, 285
impulsive insanities 20
folie circulaire 179, 180
katatonia 186, 188, 190
insanity due to brain lesions 132
insanity due to :—
Indian hemp 197, 200, 201, 202
cocaine 224
chloroform and ether 225
phthisis 291
malaria 291
syphilis 298
Mr. Justice Stephens' definition of criminal responsibility .. 20
delusions 48
eroticism 52
expert evidence .. 21
feigned insanity .. 23
hallucinations .. 46
home or asylum treatment 2
decision lies with relatives 2
attendants .. 2
home treatment requires no certification 3
impulsiveness, its origin and importance 51
menstruation and .. 20
neurasthenia and 113, 114
menstruation and insanity .. 20, 306
neurasthenic delusional psychoses 122

Pages.

stupor 49
testamentary capacity 25
transfer of lunatics to England 14
Traumatic insanity :—
its medico-legal importance .. 133, 136
ætiology 133
symptoms, physical 134
mental 135
diagnosis 136
prognosis 136
treatment 137
words of advice to the young practitioner 24
Medico-social duties .. 27
Medulla, cerebral, changes in 78
Megalomania (*see* Delusional Insanity).
Melancholia, acute 40, 142
definition 142
ætiology 143
symptoms, prodromal 143
physical 143
nervous 145
mental 145
diagnosis 147
treatment 147
drugs in 148
prognosis 148
Melancholia, Chronic (*see* Chronic Metabolic Toxæmia).
Melancholia, excited 41, 161
ætiology 162
symptoms, prodromal 162
physical 163

Pages.
mental 163
diagnosis 164
treatment 165
prognosis 165
Memory 53, 73
Menstruation and insanity 67, 306
Menstruation and criminal responsibility .. 20
Menstrual derangements in the insane 316
Mental enfeeblement 44-50
Mentalisation, derangements of 45-59
origin of .. 72
Mercurial poisoning, insanity due to .. 44-226
Metabolic toxæmias 30—40
Micro-organisms in the blood of insanes .. 31, 63, 92
Micro-organismal diseases in the insane 312
"Mittens" as a means of restraint 328
Monomania (*see* Delusional Insanity).
Morphia, indulgence in .. 220
insanity due to 44, 221
symptoms,
physical .. 221
mental .. 222
diagnosis .. 222
treatment .. 223
prognosis .. 223
"Mudeaters" 283
Myxœdema, insanity due to 149
ætiology 149

Pages.
symptoms, physical 149
mental .. 150
diagnosis 151
pathology 151
treatment 151
prognosis 152

N

Narcotics (*see* Hypnotics).
Nasal tube, feeding by .. 323
Nerve-cells (*see* Degenerations of).
Nervous system in insanity 69
Nervous diseases frequently complicated by mental disease 44
Neurasthenia 104
definition 104
ætiology 104
symptoms, physical .. 105
neuro-muscular asthenia 105
insomnia 106
mental depression .. 107
headache 108
rachialgia (pains in the back) 109
cardiac disturbances 109
digestive troubles .. 110
mental 112
dominant ideas and conceptions 113
motormental agitation 113
anxiety and obsessions 114
"délire de toucher et de doute" .. 114
diagnosis 115
treatment 116
hygienic 116

Pages.

dietetic 117
moral 118
therapeutic 119
hydrotherapeutic .. 120
drugs 120
prognosis 121

Neurasthenic psychoses .. 121
Neuroglia, degenerations of 81
Non-toxic causes of insanity 36
Nutrition of the body and insanity 68

O

Œdema of the extremities 64, 129
Œsophageal tube, feeding by 322
Old Maids Insanity (*see* Delusional Insanity).
Opium as a cause of Insanity 219
as a sedative in .. 334
Ovarian Insanity (*see* Delusional Insanity).
Ovaries in relation to insanity 68

P

Paraldehyde as a sedative 59, 334
in exhaustion insanity .. 131
in acute melancholia .. 148
in acute mania 174
in folie circulaire .. 181

Pages

in katatonia 187
in insanity due to Indian hemp .. 203
to alcohol .. 209

Paraldehyde habit 44, 225
Paranoia (*see* Delusional Insanity).
Paresis of the voluntary muscles 71
Pathology, general 74 to 92
Persecution, delusions of 48
Perspiration, excessive, in insanity .. 69, 129
Petit Mal (*see* Epilepsy).
Phthisis in the insane 64, 313
insanity due to .. 289
mental symptoms .. 290
diagnosis 291
treatment 291
prognosis 291

Physical symptoms of insanity .. .. 60 to 72
alimentary 60
circulatory 64
hæmopoietic .. 61
integumentary .. 65
nervous 69
reproductive .. 67
respiratory 64
urinary 66
vasomotor and nutritional 68

Pia mater, pathological changes in 76
Pneumonia and the insane 313
Pregnancy, insanity due to 306

Pages.

Prodromal symptoms and their importance .. 320
Prophylaxis in general treatment 320
Psychoses peculiar to India 98
Puerperal insanity 19, 40, 176
Puerperium, mania after 175
Pulse rates in insanity .. 64
Pupils in insanity .. 70
in G. P. I. 249

R

Rachialgia (*see* Neurasthenia).
Reflexes, superficial and deep, and organic .. 71
in acute melancholia 145
in excited melancholia 163
in acute mania .. 170
in folie circulaire .. 179
in katatonia .. 185, 188
in hebephrenia .. 194
in morphinism .. 221
in idiots 262
Religious instinct in insanity 52
Reproductive system and insanity 67
Respiratory system and insanity 64
Restraint, modes of applying 326
the padded room .. 326
the sheet 327
the strait waistcoat 327
the "Mittens" .. 328
Dr. Wolffe's "protective bed" .. 329

Pages.

Rheumatic fever, insanity due to 296
treatment 297
prognosis 298

S

Salivation in the insane .. 69
Salvarsan in G. P. I. .. 256
in syphilitic insanity 302
Sanity, certificates of .. 14
Sedatives 333
Self-control 50
Sensation in insanity .. 69
Sensibility in acute melancholia 145
in excited melancholia 163
in acute mania .. 170
in folie circulaire .. 179
in katatonia .. 185
in hebephrenia .. 194
in insanity due to Indian hemp .. 201
in alcoholic insanity .. 214
in morphinism .. 221
in G. P. I. .. 249, 251
Sensory hallucinations .. 48
Septicæmia and puerperal insanity 176
Serumtherapy .. 74, 331
Sexual desire in the insane 52
Shah Daula's mice 99, 268, 274
Skin in the insane .. 65
Skullcap, changes in, in insanity 75
Sleep 56, 72
Sleeplessness 57
Smell, hallucinations of 47

Pages.

Speech, derangements of,
  in insanity 53
    origin of 73
Status epilepticus .. 234
Stupor 49
Sulphonal as an hypnotic 59, 336
    in exhaustion insanity 131
    in acute melancholia 148
    in folie circulaire .. 181
    in katatonia .. 187, 191
    in hebephrenia .. 196
    in insanity due to Indian hemp .. 203
    in G. P. I. 255
Sunstroke, mental derangement due to .. 134, 292
Syphilis, insanity due to 298
  Savage's classification of 299
    true cerebral syphilis 301
    treatment 302
    prognosis 303

T

Taste, hallucinations of .. 47
Temperature in the insane 68, 83
    in acute melancholia 144
    in delusional insanity 154, 155
    in excited melancholia 163
    in acute mania .. 169
    in folie circulaire .. 178
    in katatonia 186—188
    in hebephrenia .. 194
    in epilepsy 230
    in G. P. I. 250
Temperatures, subnormal, in the insane 325

Pages.

Terebene, subcutaneous injection of 312
Testicles, their relations with insanity 68
Testamentary capacity 25
Thyroid gland and insanity 40, 61
Thyroid poisoning, insanity due to 44, 227
Thyroid treatment 62, 337
Tongue, furred 61
    tremors of, in alcoholism 216
    jerking of, in G. P. I. 216
Toxic causes of Insanity:—
    Macpherson's classification of 30
    Metabolic toxines .. 30, 40
    Bacterial toxines .. 30, 40
    Drugs, etc. 30
Transfer of lunatics to other asylums 10
Transfer of lunatics to England 14
Trauma, insanity due to 133
    ætiology 133
    symptoms, physical 134
      mental 135
    diagnosis 136
    medico-legal importance .. 133—136
    prognosis 136
    treatment 137
Treatment, general, of insanity 320
Trional as an hypnotic .. 59, 131, 334

Pages.

Tube-feeding, nasal .. 322
  œsophageal 322
Tumour of the brain and insanity 286

U

Ulcers in the insane .. 311
Upbringing of neurotic children .. 28, 321
  of idiots and imbeciles 275
Urea (*see* Urinary Excretion).
Urinary excretion in the insane 66, 67
  in acute melancholia 144
  in delusional insanity 154, 155
  in acute mania .. 169
  in folie circulaire .. 179
  in alcoholic insanity 213
  in epilepsy .. 230, 231

Pages.

Uterus in puerperal insanity 176

V

Vaccines in insanity .. 92
Valvular lesions of the heart, insanity due to .. 64, 298
Vasomotor disturbances in insanity .. 64, 68
Veronal as a sedative .. 131, 337
Volition .. 52, 73
Vomiting in the insane .. 61

W

Will (*see* Volition).
Wills, making of (*see* Testamentary Capacity).
Writing in the insane .. 54
  in imbeciles 278
Wounds in the insane .. 311